D0472915

The Nursing Assistant's Handbook

By Hartman Publishing, Inc.
with Jetta Fuzy, RN, MS

SECOND EDITION

Nursing Department
Sierra College
5000 Rocklin Road
Rocklin, CA 95677

JUN 2 0 2007

Credits

MANAGING EDITOR
Susan Alvare

COVER AND INTERIOR DESIGNER
Kirsten Browne

ILLUSTRATORS
Thaddeus Castillo/Robert Christopher

PAGE LAYOUT
Thaddeus Castillo

PHOTOGRAPHY
Art Clifton/Dick Ruddy/Pat Berrett

PROOFREADERS
Suzanne Wegner
Holly Day
Mike Marlow

SALES/MARKETING
Debbie Rinker/Kay Kreiner/Ernest Culver

CUSTOMER SERVICE
Kim Williams/Erin Herridge

Special Thanks

We are so appreciative of our insightful and
wonderful reviewers:

Lori Dunbar, RN
Springdale, AR

Sally Lyle, RN
Rock Hill, SC

Kimberly D. Powell, RN
Fayetteville, AR

Jean P. Stanhagen, RN, BSN
Bethel Park, PA

Kathie Zimmerman, RN
Harrisburg, PA

Many wonderful and informative photos came from
the following sources:
Lee Penner of Penner Tubs
The Briggs Corporation
North Coast Medical, Inc.
Innovative Products Unlimited
Dr. Frederick Miller
Dr. Jeffrey T. Behr
VANCARE, Inc.
Merry Walker Corporation
Dr. Tamara D. Fishman and The Wound Care
Institute, Inc.
RG Medical Diagnostics of Southfield, MI
Detecto
Lenjoy Medical Engineering

Copyright Information

© 2007 by Hartman Publishing, Inc.
8529 Indian School Road, NE
Albuquerque, New Mexico 87112
(505) 291-1274
web: www.**hartman**online.com
e-mail: orders@**hartman**online.com

All rights reserved. No part of this book may be repro-
duced, in any form or by any means, without permission in writing from the publisher.

ISBN-10 1-888343-91-5
ISBN-13 978-1-8883-4391-5

NOTICE TO READERS
Though the guidelines and procedures contained in this text are based on consultations with healthcare professionals, they should not be considered absolute recommendations. The instructor and readers should follow employer, local, state, and federal guidelines concerning healthcare practices. These guidelines change, and it is the reader's responsibility to be aware of these changes and of the policies and procedures of her or his healthcare facility.

The publisher, author, editors, and reviewers cannot accept any responsibility for errors or omissions or for any conse-quences from application of the information in this book and make no warranty, expressed or implied, with respect to the contents of the book. The Publisher does not warrant or guarantee any of the products described herein or perform any analysis in connection with any of the product information contained herein.

GENDER USAGE
This textbook utilizes the pronouns "he," "his," "she," and "hers" interchangeably to denote healthcare team members and residents.

table of contents

𝒫 denotes a practical procedure

six

Basic Nursing Skills 118

seven

Nutrition and Hydration 156

eight
Common, Chronic, and Acute Conditions   174

nine
Rehabilitation and Restorative Services   204

ten
Caring for Yourself   219

Welcome to The Nursing Assistant's Handbook

We have divided this book into ten chapters and assigned each chapter its own colored tab, which you'll see at the top of every page. Within that tab, you'll find the name of the section that is being taught.

Unit 6: Describe and demonstrate infection control practices

Everything you will learn in this book is organized around learning objectives. A learning objective is a specific piece of knowledge or a very specific skill.

Making an occupied bed

All care procedures will have numbered steps. Underneath each step is the reason why it is important for you to perform this step.

This icon is found at the end of some procedures. It points out common errors that students make when they are tested on this skill during a certification exam.

This icon emphasizes Residents' Rights. These are very important rights for residents who live in nursing homes. They are the law and must always be followed.

State agencies perform inspections on nursing homes on a regular basis. These inspections are called surveys. This sign shows you what facilities are often cited for during surveys.

The blood vessels **constrict**, or close, when the outside temperature is too cold.

You'll find bold **key terms** throughout the text. These are important terms you need to know.

Guidelines:
Hearing Impairment

Common Disorders, Guidelines, and Observing and Reporting are colored red for easy reference.

one

Long-Term Care and the Nursing Assistant's Role

Unit 1. Compare long-term care to other healthcare settings

Welcome to the world of health care. Health care happens in many places. Nursing assistants work in many of these settings. In each setting, similar tasks will be performed. However, each setting is also unique.

This textbook will focus on settings that provide long-term care. **Long-term care** (**LTC**) is for persons who need 24-hour care and help for conditions that are long-term. Other terms for long-term care facilities are nursing homes, nursing facilities, skilled nursing facilities, or extended care facilities. The people who live in these facilities may be disabled and/or elderly. They may come from hospitals or other facilities. Some will have a terminal illness. **Terminal** means the person is expected to die from the illness. Some people come to nursing homes for conditions that require care for six months or longer. Other people come for short stays. Some people recover and return to their homes or to assisted living facilities.

Most conditions seen in nursing homes are **chronic**. This means they last a long period of time, even a lifetime. Chronic conditions include physical disabilities, heart disease, stroke, and dementia. (You will learn more about these disorders and diseases in chapter 8.) Working in a nursing home, you will form relationships with residents for longer periods of time than in other healthcare settings.

The person for whom you will care may be called a "resident," "patient," or "client." The person's diagnosis, or medical condition, will vary. The stages of an illness or disease affect how sick people are and how much care they will need. The job of the nursing assistant will also vary. This is due to the person's different symptoms, abilities, and needs. This book focuses on the role of the nursing assistant in the nursing home. While people live in this facility, it is their home. This is why the people who live there are called residents. This is how this book will refer to the people for whom you will be providing care. The facility will be a resident's home until he or she returns home, moves to another place, or dies.

Other types of healthcare settings are:

Acute care is performed in hospitals and ambulatory surgical centers. Persons are admitted for short stays for surgery or diseases. Acute care offers 24-hour skilled care for temporary, but serious, illnesses or injuries (Fig. 1-1). **Skilled care** is medically necessary care given by a skilled nurse or therapist. This care is available 24 hours a day. It is ordered by a doctor, and involves a treatment plan.

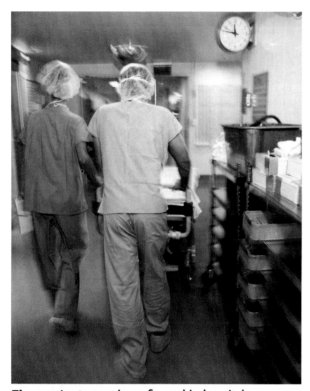

Fig. 1-1. Acute care is performed in hospitals.

Subacute care can be found in either a hospital or a nursing home. The residents need more care and observation than some long-term care facilities can offer. The cost is usually less than a hospital but more than long-term care.

Outpatient care is usually given for less than 24 hours. It is for people who have had treatments or surgery that require short-term skilled care.

Rehabilitation is care provided by a specialist. This is a person trained to provide special care. Physical, occupational, and speech therapists restore or improve function after an illness or injury.

In **assisted living** residents need some help with daily care, such as showers and meals. They may also need assistance with medications. Staff give whatever daily care the resident needs. Residents do not usually require skilled care.

Home health care is provided in a person's home. Home care includes many of the services offered in other settings (Fig. 1-2).

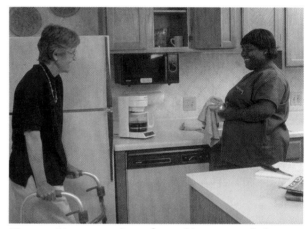

Fig. 1-2. Home care is performed in a person's home.

Adult daycare is given at a facility during daytime work hours. Generally, adult daycare cares for people who need some help but are not seriously ill or disabled. A center may be a part of another facility, or it may stand alone. The daily fee is usually much less than the cost of a long-term care facility.

Hospice care is for people who have six months or less to live. Hospice workers give physical and emotional care and comfort. They also support families. Hospice care can take place in facilities or in homes.

Unit 2. Describe a typical long-term care facility

A long-term care facility may provide only skilled nursing care. It may also offer assisted living, dementia care, or even subacute care. Some facilities offer specialized care. Others provide care for all types of residents. The typical long-term care facility offers personal care for all residents and focused care for residents with special needs. When specialized care is offered, the employees may have special training. Residents with similar conditions may be placed in units together.

For-profit companies or nonprofit organizations can own facilities. More information about the care team and how the members work together is found later in the chapter.

Unit 3. Explain Medicare and Medicaid

The Centers for Medicare & Medicaid Services (CMS), formerly the Health Care Finance Administration (HCFA), is a federal agency within the U.S. Department of Health and Human Services (Fig. 1-3). CMS runs two national healthcare programs, Medicare and Medicaid. They both help pay for health care and health insurance for millions of Americans. CMS has many other responsibilities as well.

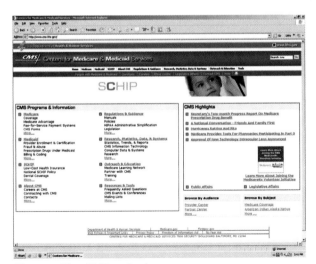

Fig. 1-3. The CMS web site.

Medicare is a health insurance program for people who are 65 years or older. It also covers people younger than 65 but who are dis-

abled or ill and cannot work. Medicare has two parts: Part A and Part B, which cover different medical services. Medicare covers a percentage of a person's healthcare costs. Medicare will only pay for care it determines to be medically necessary.

Medicaid is a medical assistance program for low-income people. It is funded by both the federal government and each state. Eligibility is determined by income and special circumstances. People must qualify for this program.

Medicare and Medicaid pay long-term care facilities a fixed amount for services. This amount is based on the resident's needs upon admission.

Unit 4. Describe the role of the nursing assistant

Nursing assistants can have many different titles. Nurse aide, unlicensed assistive personnel, and certified nursing assistant are some examples. This book will use the term "nursing assistant." The nursing assistant (NA) performs delegated or assigned nursing tasks, such as taking a resident's temperature. A nursing assistant also provides personal care, such as bathing residents.

Other nursing assistant duties include:

- feeding residents

- helping residents with toileting and elimination needs

- assisting residents to move safely around the facility

- keeping residents' living areas neat and clean

- encouraging residents to eat and drink (Fig. 1-4)

- caring for supplies and equipment

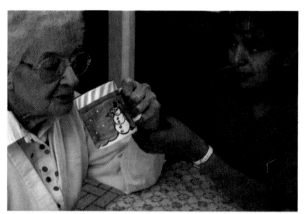

Fig. 1-4. Assisting a resident with drinking will be one of your duties.

- helping to dress residents
- making beds
- giving backrubs
- helping residents with mouth care

📄 *Nursing assistants are not allowed to give medications. Nurses are responsible for giving medications. Some states allow nursing assistants to give medications after receiving special training. Examples of other tasks that nursing assistants are generally not allowed to do are inserting/removing tubes, changing sterile dressings, and giving tube feedings.*

Nursing assistants spend more time with residents than other team members do. They act as the "eyes and ears" of the team. Observing changes in a resident's condition and reporting them is a very important role. You will also write down important information about the resident (Fig. 1-5). This is called **charting**.

Nursing assistants are part of a team of health professionals. The team includes physicians, nurses, social workers, therapists, dietitians, and specialists. The resident's family is part of the team. Everyone, including the resident, works closely together. Goals include helping residents recover from illnesses or do as much as possible for themselves.

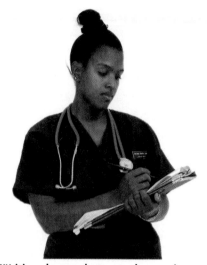

Fig. 1-5. Writing down what you observe is one of the most important duties you'll have.

Unit 5. Describe the care team and the chain of command

Residents have different needs and problems. This means that people with different kinds of education and experience help care for them (Fig. 1-6). This group is the **care team**. Members of the care team include:

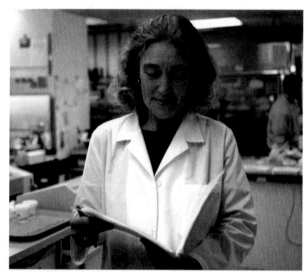

Fig. 1-6. The care team is made up of many different professionals.

Registered Nurse (RN). An RN is a licensed professional who has completed two to four years of education. The nurse assesses residents' status, monitors progress, and provides skilled nursing care. The nurse gives treatments, including drug therapies, as prescribed by a doctor. The nurse assigns and supervises your daily care of residents. The nurse also writes and develops care plans. A **care plan** is created for each resident. It helps the resident achieve his or her goals. The care plan outlines the steps and tasks the care team must perform.

Licensed Practical Nurse (LPN) or Licensed Vocational Nurse (LVN). A LPN/LVN is a licensed professional who has completed one to two years of education. A LPN/LVN passes medications and gives treatments. LPNs may supervise daily care of residents.

Physician or Doctor (MD or DO). A doctor diagnoses disease or disability and prescribes treatment. Doctors attend four-year medical schools after receiving a bachelor's degree (Fig. 1-7). ("DO" stands for "doctor of osteopathic medicine.")

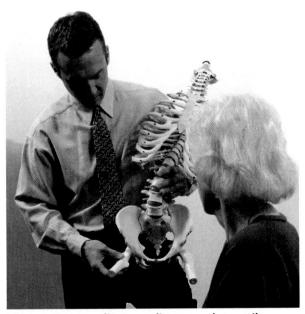

Fig. 1-7. Doctors diagnose disease and prescribe treatment.

Physical Therapist (PT). The physical therapist gives therapy in the form of heat, cold, massage, ultrasound, electricity, and exercise to people with muscle, bone, and joint problems. Goals of physical therapy are improving blood circulation, healing, regaining mobility, and easing pain. For example, a PT helps a person to safely use a walker, cane, or wheelchair (Fig. 1-8).

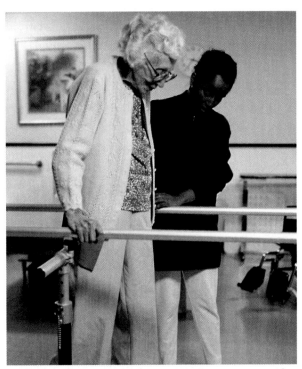

Fig. 1-8. A physical therapist will help restore specific abilities.

Occupational Therapist (OT). An occupational therapist helps residents learn to compensate for disabilities. An OT helps residents be able to do **activities of daily living (ADL)**. ADLs are personal daily care tasks. They include bathing, dressing, caring for teeth and hair, toileting, and eating and drinking. For example, an OT teaches a person to use a special spoon so that she can feed herself.

Speech Language Pathologist (SLP). A speech language pathologist or speech therapist helps residents with speech and swallowing problems. For example, after a stroke, a person may not be able to talk. An SLP may use a picture board to have the person communicate thirst or pain. An SLP also evaluates a person's ability to swallow food and drink.

Registered Dietitian (RDT). A registered dietitian or nutritionist creates special diets for residents with special needs. Special diets can improve health and help manage illness.

Medical Social Worker (MSW). A medical social worker helps residents with social needs. For example, an MSW helps residents find compatible roommates. He or she also helps with support services. These include obtaining clothing and personal items if the family is not involved or does not visit frequently. An MSW may book appointments and arrange transportation.

Activities Director. The activities director plans activities, such as bingo or special performances. This helps residents socialize and stay physically and mentally active.

Nursing Assistant (NA) or Certified Nursing Assistant (CNA). The nursing assistant does delegated or assigned tasks, such as taking a resident's temperature. NAs also give personal care, such as bathing residents and helping with toileting. NAs must have at least 75 hours of training. In many states, training exceeds 100 hours.

Resident and Resident's Family. The resident is an important member of the care team. The resident has the right to make decisions about his or her own care. The resident helps plan care and makes choices. The resident's family may also be involved in these decisions. The family is a great source of information. They know the resident's personal preferences, history, diet, rituals, and routines.

All members of the care team should focus on the resident. The team revolves around the resident and his or her condition, treatment, and progress. Without the resident, there is no team.

As a nursing assistant, you will follow instructions given to you by a nurse. The nurse acts on the instructions of a doctor or other care team member. This is called the **chain of command**. It describes the line of authority in the facility. The chain of command coordinates care to provide the best care for residents. It also protects you and your employer from liability. **Liability** is a legal term. It means a person can be held responsible for harming someone else. Example: Something you did for a resident harmed him. However, what you did was assigned to you. It was done according to policy and procedure. Then, you may not be liable, or responsible, for hurting the resident. If you do something not assigned to you and it harms a resident, you could be held responsible. That is why it is important to follow instructions and know the chain of command (Fig. 1-9).

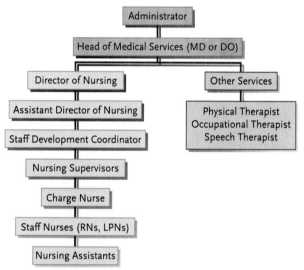

Fig. 1-9. The chain of command describes the line of authority in a facility.

Nursing assistants must understand what they can and cannot do. This is so that you do not harm a resident or involve yourself or your employer in a lawsuit. Some states certify that a nursing assistant is qualified to work. However, nursing assistants are not licensed healthcare providers. Everything you do in your job is assigned to you by a licensed healthcare professional. You work under the authority of another person's license. That is why these professionals will show great interest in what you do and how you do it.

Every state grants the right to do various jobs in health care through licensing. Examples include nursing, medicine, or physical therapy. All members of the care team work under each profession's "scope of practice." A **scope of practice** defines the things you are allowed to do and how to do them correctly.

Unit 6. Define policies, procedures, and professionalism

All facilities must have manuals outlining policies and procedures. A **policy** is a course of action to be followed. A very basic policy is that healthcare information must remain confidential. A **procedure** is a method, or way, of doing something. A facility will have a procedure for reporting information about residents. The procedure explains what form to complete, when and how often to fill it out, and to whom it is given. You will be told where to locate a list of policies and procedures that all staff are expected to follow.

Common policies at long-term care facilities include the following:

- All resident information must remain confidential.
- The care plan must always be followed.
- Nursing assistants should not do tasks not included in the job description.
- Nursing assistants must report important events or changes in residents to a nurse.
- Personal problems must not be discussed with the resident or the resident's family.
- Nursing assistants should not take money or gifts from residents or their families.

- Nursing assistants must be on time for work and dependable.

Your employer will have policies and procedures for every resident care situation. Written procedures may seem long and complicated, but each step is important. Become familiar with your facility's policies and procedures.

Professional means having to do with work or a job. The opposite of professional is **personal**. It refers to your life outside your job, such as your family, friends, and home life. **Professionalism** is behaving properly on the job. It includes how you dress, the words you use, and what you talk about. It also means being on time, completing tasks, and reporting to the nurse. Professionalism is also following the care plan, making careful observations, and always reporting accurately. Following policies and procedures is an important part of professionalism.

Residents, coworkers, and supervisors respect employees who are professional. Professionalism helps you keep your job. It also helps you earn promotions and raises.

A professional relationship with a resident includes:

- keeping a positive attitude
- doing only the assigned tasks you are trained to do
- keeping all residents' information confidential
- being polite and cheerful, even if you are not in a good mood (Fig. 1-10)
- not discussing your personal problems
- not using profanity, even if a resident does
- listening to the resident
- calling a resident "Mr.," "Mrs.," "Ms.," or "Miss," or by the name he or she prefers

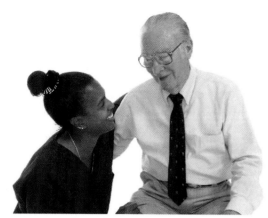

Fig. 1-10. Being polite and cheerful is something that will be expected of you.

- always explaining the care you will provide before providing it

- following practices, such as handwashing, to protect yourself and residents

A professional relationship with an employer includes:

- completing tasks efficiently

- always following all policies and procedures

- always documenting and reporting carefully and correctly

- communicating problems with residents or tasks

- reporting anything that keeps you from completing duties

- asking questions when you do not know or understand something

- taking directions or criticism without getting upset

- being clean and neatly dressed and groomed (Fig. 1-11)

- always being on time

- telling your employer if you cannot report for work

- following the chain of command

- participating in education programs

- being a positive role model

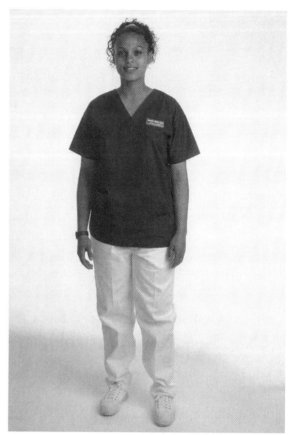

Fig. 1-11. Keeping your hair neatly tied back and wearing a clean uniform are examples of professional behavior.

The best nursing assistants have these qualities:

- **Compassion.** Being **compassionate** is being caring, concerned, empathetic, and understanding. **Empathy** means entering into the feelings of others. Compassionate people are also sympathetic. **Sympathy** means sharing in the feelings and difficulties of others.

- **Honesty.** An honest person tells the truth and can be trusted.

- **Tact.** **Tact** is the ability to understand what is proper and appropriate when dealing with others. It is the ability to speak and act without offending others.

- **Conscientiousness.** People who are **conscientious** always try to do their best. They are always alert, observant, accurate, and responsible.

- **Dependability**. Nursing assistants must make and keep commitments. You must get to work on time. You must skillfully do tasks and help your peers when they need it.

- **Respect**. Being respectful means valuing other people's individuality. This includes their age, religion, culture, feelings, practices, and beliefs.

- **Lack of prejudice**. You will work with people from different backgrounds. Give each resident quality care regardless of age, gender, sexual orientation, religion, race, ethnicity, or condition.

- **Tolerance**. You may not like or agree with things that your residents have done. However, your job is to provide care, not to judge them. Put aside your opinions. See each resident as an individual who needs your care.

Unit 7. List examples of legal and ethical behavior and explain Residents' Rights

Ethics and laws guide behavior. **Ethics** is the knowledge of right and wrong. An ethical person has a sense of duty toward others. He always tries to do what is right. **Laws** are rules set by the government to protect people and help them live peacefully together. Ethics and laws are very important in health care. They protect people receiving care. They guide those giving care. NAs and other team members follow a code of ethics. They must know the laws that apply to their jobs.

Examples of legal and ethical behavior by nursing assistants include the following:

- being honest at all times

- protecting residents' privacy

- keeping resident and staff information confidential

- reporting abuse or suspected abuse of a resident or assisting a resident in reporting abuse

- following the care plan and assignments

- not performing tasks outside your scope of practice

- reporting all resident observations and incidents

- documenting accurately and on time

- following rules on safety and infection control (chapter 2)

- not accepting gifts or tips

- never becoming personally or sexually involved with residents or family members

Due to reports of poor care and abuse in nursing homes, the U.S. government passed the **Omnibus Budget Reconciliation Act (OBRA)** in 1987. It has been updated several times.

OBRA set minimum standards for nursing assistant training. NAs must complete at least 75 hours of training. NAs must also pass a competency evaluation (testing program) before they can be employed. They must attend regular in-service education to keep skills updated.

OBRA requires that states keep a current list of nursing assistants in a state registry. OBRA sets guidelines for minimum staff requirements. It specifies the minimum services that nursing homes must provide. Another important part of OBRA is the resident assessment requirements. OBRA requires complete assessments on every resident. The assessment forms are the same for every facility.

OBRA made major changes in the survey process. You first learned about surveys in the beginning pages of this book. The results from surveys are available to the public and posted in the facility.

OBRA also identified important rights for residents in nursing homes. **Residents' Rights** relate to how residents must be treated while living in a facility. They are an ethical code of conduct for healthcare workers. These rights include:

Quality of life: Residents have the right to the best care available. Dignity, choice, and independence are important parts of quality of life.

Services and activities to maintain a high level of wellness: Residents must receive the correct care. Their care should keep them as healthy as possible every day. Health should not decline as a direct result of the facility's care.

The right to be fully informed regarding rights and services: Residents must be told what care and services are available. They must be told the charges for each service. They must be aware of all their legal rights. Legal rights must be explained in a language they can understand. This includes being given a written copy of their rights. They have the right to be notified in advance of any change of room or roommate. They have the right to communicate with someone who speaks their language. They have the right to assistance for any sensory impairment. Blindness is one type of sensory impairment.

The right to participate in their own care: Residents have the right to participate in planning their treatment, care, and discharge. Residents have the right to refuse medication, treatment, and restraints. They have the right to be told of changes in their condition. They have the right to review

their medical record. Informed consent is a concept that goes along with this. A person has the legal and ethical right to direct what happens to his or her body. Doctors also have an ethical duty to involve the person in his or her health care. **Informed consent** is the process in which a person, with the help of a doctor, makes informed decisions about his or her health care.

The right to make independent choices: Residents can make choices about their doctors, care, and treatments. They can make personal decisions, such as what to wear and how to spend their time. They can join in community activities.

The right to privacy and confidentiality: Residents can expect privacy with care given. Their medical and personal information cannot be shared with anyone but the care team. Residents have the right to private, unrestricted communication with anyone.

The right to dignity, respect, and freedom: Residents must be respected and treated with dignity by caregivers. Residents cannot be abused in any way.

The right to security of possessions: Residents' personal possessions must be safe at all times. They cannot be taken or used by anyone without a resident's permission.

Rights during transfers and discharges: Location changes must be made safely and with the resident's knowledge and consent. Residents have the right to stay in a facility unless a transfer or discharge is needed.

The right to complain: Residents have the right to complain without fear of punishment. Nursing homes must work quickly to try to resolve complaints.

The right to visits: Residents have the right to have visits from family, doctors, groups and others (Fig. 1-12).

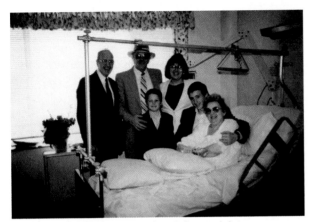

Fig. 1-12. Residents have the right to visitors.

Protect your residents' rights in these ways:

- Never abuse a resident physically, emotionally, verbally, or sexually.

- Watch for and report any signs of abuse or neglect.

- Call the resident by the name he or she prefers.

- Involve residents in your planning.

- Always explain a procedure to a resident before performing it.

- Do not unnecessarily expose a resident while giving care.

- Respect a resident's refusal of care. However, report the refusal to the nurse immediately.

- Tell the nurse if a resident has questions about the goals of care or the care plan.

- Be truthful when documenting care.

- Do not talk or gossip about residents.

- Knock and ask for permission before entering a resident's room.

- Do not accept gifts or money (Fig. 1-13).

- Do not open a resident's mail or look through his belongings.

- Respect residents' personal possessions.

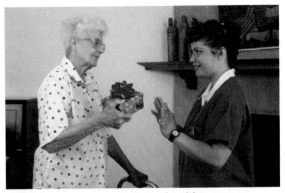

Fig. 1-13. Nursing assistants should not accept money or gifts because it is unprofessional and leads to conflict.

- Report observations about a resident's condition or care.

- Help resolve disputes by reporting to the nurse.

RA *A Residents' Council is a group of residents who meet regularly to discuss issues related to the nursing home. This Council gives residents a voice in facility operations. Topics of discussion may include facility policies, decisions regarding activities, concerns, and problems. The Residents' Council offers residents a chance to provide suggestions on improving the quality of care. Council executives are elected by residents. Family members are invited to attend meetings with or on behalf of residents. Staff may participate in this process when invited by Council members.*

Abuse is purposely causing physical, mental, or emotional pain or injury to someone. Shoving a resident is an example of physical abuse. Purposely embarrassing a resident is an example of emotional or psychological abuse.

Neglect is harming the person in your care physically, mentally, or emotionally by failing to give needed care. Deliberately ignoring a resident is an example of neglect.

Physical abuse is any treatment, intentional or not, that causes harm to a person's body. This includes slapping, bruising, cutting, burning, physically restraining, pushing, shoving, or even rough handling.

Sexual abuse is forcing a person to perform or participate in sexual acts.

Psychological or **mental abuse** is emotionally harming a person by threatening, scaring, humiliating, intimidating, isolating, insulting, or treating him or her as a child. It includes verbal abuse. **Verbal abuse** is oral or written words, pictures, or gestures that threaten, embarrass, or insult a resident.

Financial abuse is stealing, taking advantage of, or improperly using the money, property, or other assets of another.

Assault happens when a person is threatened and feels fearful that he or she will be touched without their permission. Telling a resident that she will be slapped if she does not stop yelling is an example.

Battery means a person is actually touched without his or her permission. An example is a nursing assistant hitting or pushing a resident. It is also physical abuse. Forcing a resident to eat a meal is also battery.

Domestic violence is abuse by spouses, intimate partners, or family members. It can be physical, sexual, or emotional. The victim can be a woman, man, elderly person, or a child.

Workplace violence is abuse of staff by residents or other staff members. It can be verbal, physical, or sexual. This includes improper touching and discussion about sexual subjects.

False imprisonment is the unlawful restraint of someone which affects the per-son's freedom of movement. Both the threat of being physically restrained and actually being physically restrained are false imprisonment. Not allowing a resident to leave the building is also false imprisonment.

Involuntary seclusion is confinement or separation from others in a certain area. It is done without consent or against one's will.

Sexual harassment is any unwelcome sexual advance or behavior that creates an intimidating, hostile or offensive working environment. Requests for sexual favors, unwanted touching, and other acts of a sexual nature are examples of sexual harassment.

Substance abuse is the use of legal or illegal drugs, cigarettes, or alcohol in a way that harms oneself or others.

Negligence means the failure to provide the proper care for a resident that results in unintended injury. Examples of negligence are:

- You do not notice that your resident's dentures do not fit properly. Because they do not, he is not eating well. He becomes malnourished.

- You forget to lock a resident's wheelchair before transferring her. She falls and is injured.

If you see or suspect abuse or neglect, you are legally required to report it.

Observing and Reporting Abuse and Neglect

These are "suspicious injuries." They should be reported:

- poisoning or traumatic injury

- teeth marks

- belt buckle or strap marks

- old and new bruises, contusions and welts

- fractures, dislocation
- burns of unusual shape and in unusual locations, cigarette burns, scalding burns
- scratches and puncture wounds
- scalp tenderness and patches of missing hair
- swelling in the face, broken teeth, nasal discharge

Signs that could indicate abuse include:

- yelling obscenities
- fear, apprehension, fear of being alone
- poor self-control
- constant pain
- threatening to hurt others
- complaints of anxiety
- withdrawal or apathy (Fig. 1-14)

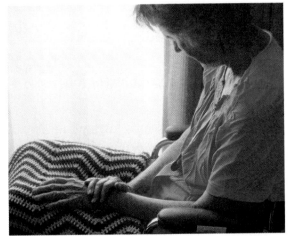

Fig. 1-14. Withdrawing from others is an important change to report.

- alcohol or drug abuse
- agitation or anxiety, signs of stress
- low self-esteem
- mood changes, confusion, disorientation
- private conversations are not allowed, or the family member/caregiver is present during all conversations

Signs that could indicate neglect include:

- pressure sores (See chapter 5 for more information.)

- body not clean
- body lice
- unanswered call lights
- soiled bedding or incontinence briefs not being changed
- poorly-fitting clothing
- refusal of care
- unmet needs relating to hearing aids, glasses, etc.
- weight loss
- poor appetite
- dehydration
- uneaten food
- fresh water or beverages not being passed each shift

If residents want to make a complaint of abuse, you must help them in every possible way. This includes informing them of the process and their rights.

An ombudsman can assist residents, too. An **ombudsman** is assigned by law as the legal advocate for residents. The ombudsman visits and listens to residents. He or she decides what action to take if there is a problem. Ombudsmen provide an ongoing presence in nursing homes. They monitor care and conditions (Fig. 1-15).

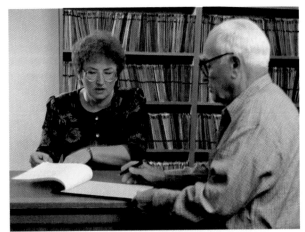

Fig. 1-15. An ombudsman is a legal advocate for residents.

To respect **confidentiality** means to keep private things private. You will learn confidential (private) information about your residents. You may learn about health, finances, and relationships. Ethically and legally, you must protect this information. You should not tell anyone except members of the care team anything about your residents.

Congress passed the **Health Insurance Portability and Accountability Act** (**HIPAA**) in 1996. It was refined and revised in 2001 and again in 2002. One reason for this law is to keep health information private and secure. All healthcare organizations must take special steps to protect health information. They and their employees can be fined and/or imprisoned if they break rules that protect patient privacy. This applies to all healthcare providers, including doctors, nurses, nursing assistants, and all team members.

Under this law, health information must be kept private. It is called protected health information (PHI). PHI includes the patient's name, address, telephone number, social security number, e-mail address, and medical record number. Only those who must have information for care or to process records should know this information. They must protect the information. It must not become known or used by anyone else. It must be kept confidential.

NAs cannot give out any resident information to anyone not directly involved in the resident's care. For example, if a neighbor asks you how a resident is doing, reply, "I'm sorry, but I cannot share that information. It's confidential." That is the correct response to anyone who does not have a legal reason to know about the resident.

Other ways to protect residents' privacy are:

- Make sure you are in a private area when you listen to or read your messages.

- Know with whom you are speaking on the phone. If you are not sure, get a name and number. Call back after you get approval.

- When talking to a care team member on the phone, do not use cellular phones. They can be scanned.

- Do not talk about residents in public (Fig. 1-16). Public areas include elevators, grocery stores, lounges, waiting rooms, parking garages, schools, restaurants, etc.

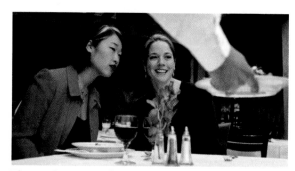

Fig. 1-16. Do not discuss residents in public places.

- Use confidential rooms for reports to other care team members.

- If you see a resident's family member or a former resident in public, be careful with your greeting. He or she may not want others to know about the family member or that he or she has been a resident.

- Do not bring family or friends to the facility to meet residents.

- Make sure nobody can see health information on your computer screen.

- Log off when not on your computer.

- Do not send confidential information in e-mails.

- Make sure fax numbers are correct before faxing information. Use a cover sheet with a confidentiality statement.

- Do not leave documents where others may see them.

- Store and file documents according to facility policy. If you find documents with a resident's information, give them to the nurse.

All healthcare workers must follow HIPAA regulations no matter where they are or what they are doing. There are serious penalties for violating these rules, including:

- Fines ranging from $100 to $250,000
- Prison sentences of up to ten years

Invasion of privacy is a legal term that means violating someone's right to privacy by exposing his or her private affairs, name, or photograph to the public without that person's consent. Discussing a resident's care or personal affairs with anyone other than your supervisor or another member of the healthcare team could be considered an invasion of privacy, which violates civil law.

Unit 8. **Explain legal aspects of the resident's medical record**

The resident's medical record is a legal document. There are legal aspects to your documentation. Careful charting is important for these four reasons:

1. It is the only way to guarantee clear and complete communication between all the members of the care team.

2. It is a legal record of every resident's treatment. Medical charts can be used in court as legal evidence.

3. Documentation protects you and your employer from liability by proving what you did.

4. Documentation gives an up-to-date record of the status and care of each resident (Fig. 1-17).

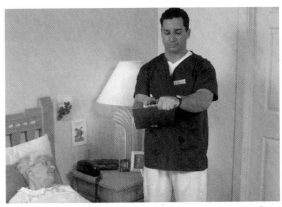

Fig. 1-17. Documentation provides important information about the resident.

Guidelines
Careful Documentation

- Write your notes immediately after the care is given. This helps you to remember important details. **Do not record care before it is done**.

- Think about what you want to say before writing. This will help you be as brief and as clear as possible.

- Write facts, not opinions.

- Write neatly. Use black ink.

- If you make a mistake, draw one line through it. Write the correct word or words. Put your initials and the date. Never erase something you have written. Never use correction fluid (Fig. 1-18).

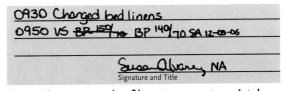

Fig. 1-18. An example of how to correct a mistake.

- Sign your full name and title. Write the correct date.

- Document as specified in the care plan. Some facilities have a "check-off" sheet for documenting care. It is also called an ADL (activities of daily living) or flow sheet.

- Facilities may want you to use the 24-hour clock, or military time, to document information. Figure 1-19 shows the 24-hour clock and the corresponding military time. To change the hours between 1:00 p.m. to 11:59 p.m. to military time, add 12 to the regular time. For example, to change 4:00 p.m. to military time, add 4 + 12. The answer is 1600 hours.

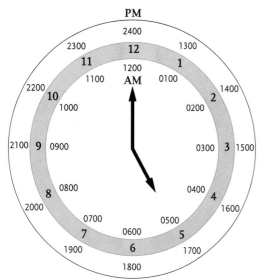

Fig. 1-19. Divisions in the 24-hour clock.

To change from military time to regular time, subtract 12. For example, to change 2200 hours to standard time, subtract 12 from 22. The answer is 10:00 p.m.

Some facilities use computers to document information. Computers record and store information. It can be retrieved when it is needed. This is faster and more accurate than writing information by hand. If your facility uses computers for documentation, you will be trained to use them. HIPAA privacy guidelines apply to computer use. Make sure nobody can see private and protected health or personal information on your computer screen. Do not share confidential information with anyone except the care team.

Unit 9. **Explain the Minimum Data Set (MDS)**

A resident assessment system was developed in 1990. It is revised periodically. It is

called the Minimum Data Set (MDS). The MDS is a detailed guide to help nurses complete resident assessments accurately. It also details what to do if resident problems are identified (Fig. 1-20). Facilities must complete the MDS for each resident within 14 days of admission and again each year. In addition, the MDS for each resident must be reviewed every three months. A new MDS must be done when there is any major change in the resident's condition.

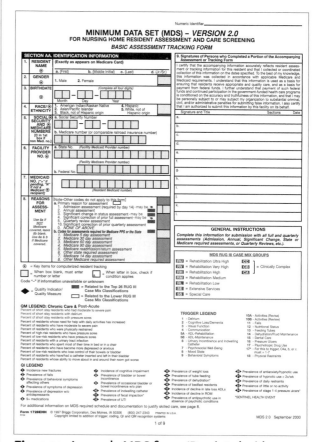

Fig. 1-20. A sample MDS form. (Reprinted with permission of the Briggs Corporation, 800-247-2343.)

The reporting you do on changes in your residents may "trigger" a needed assessment. Always report changes you notice to the nurse. They may be a sign of an illness or problem. By reporting them promptly, a new MDS assessment can be done if needed.

two

Foundations of Resident Care

Unit 1. **Understand the importance of verbal and written communications**

Effective communication is a critical part of your job. Nursing assistants must communicate with supervisors, the care team, residents, and family members. A resident's health depends on how well you communicate your observations and concerns to the nurse.

Communication is the exchange of information with others. It includes sending and receiving messages. People communicate with signs and symbols, such as words, drawings, and pictures. They also communicate by behavior.

Verbal communication uses words or sounds, spoken or written. Oral reports are an example of verbal communication. **Nonverbal communication** is communicating without using words. Examples are shaking your head or shrugging your shoulders. Nonverbal communication changes the message. Be aware of your body language and gestures when you speak (Fig. 2-1). A resident may speak a different language. You may need to use pictures or gestures to communicate.

RA *When caring for residents, always use a language they can understand or find an interpreter (someone who speaks their language). Do not speak with other staff in a different language in front of residents.*

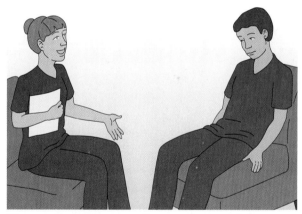

Fig. 2-1. Body language often speaks as plainly as words. Which of these people seems more interested in the conversation they are having?

Nursing assistants must be able to make brief, accurate oral and written reports to residents and staff. Good communication is needed to collect information about residents. Communicating with residents or their families gives you information that is important to the care team. This information may be written or given in oral reports from one shift to the next. Remember that all resident information is confidential. Only share information with the care team.

Your careful observations are important to the health and well-being of all residents. Deciding what to report immediately to the nurse involves critical thinking. For the NA, critical thinking is making good observations to get help for potential problems. Signs and symptoms that should be reported will be discussed in this book. In addition, anything that endangers residents should be reported immediately, including:

- falls
- chest pain
- severe headache
- trouble breathing
- abnormal pulse, respiration, or blood pressure
- change in mental status
- sudden weakness or loss of mobility
- high fever
- loss of consciousness
- change in level of consciousness
- bleeding
- change in condition
- bruises, abrasions, or other signs of abuse

When residents report symptoms, events, or feelings, have them repeat what they have said. Ask them for more information. Avoid asking questions that can be answered with a simple "yes" or "no." Instead, ask questions that ask for more detailed information. For example, asking, "Did you sleep well last night?" could easily be answered "yes" or "no." However, "Tell me about your night and how you slept" will encourage the resident to offer facts and details.

Communicating with Residents

When communicating with residents, remember to:

- *Always greet the resident by his or her preferred name.*
- *Identify yourself.*
- *Focus on the appropriate topic to be discussed.*
- *Face the resident while speaking. Avoid talking off into space.*
- *Talk with the resident while giving care.*
- *Listen and respond when the resident speaks.*
- *Praise the resident and smile often.*
- *Encourage the resident to interact with you and others.*
- *Be courteous.*
- *Always tell the resident when you are leaving the room.*

RЯ *Never refer to a resident by disrespectful terms such as "sweetie" or "honey."*

When making a report, you must collect the right information before documenting it. Facts, not opinions, are most useful to the nurse and the care team. Two kinds of factual information are needed in your reporting. **Objective information** is based on what you see, hear, touch, or smell. Objective information is collected by using the senses. **Subjective information** is something you cannot or did not observe. It is based on something that the resident reported to you that may or may not be true. An example of objective information is, "Mr. McClain is holding his head and rubbing his temples." A subjective report might be, "Mr. McClain says he has a headache." The nurse needs factual information in order to make decisions about care and treatment. Both objective and subjective reports are valuable.

Make sure what you observe and what the resident reports to you are clearly noted. In order to report accurately, you need to observe accurately. In order to observe accurately, you will use as many senses as possible to gather information (Fig. 2-2). Some examples follow the illustration.

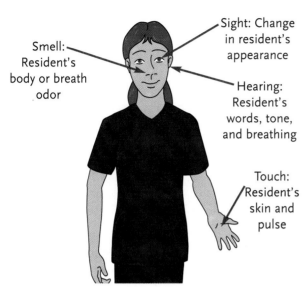

Smell: Resident's body or breath odor

Sight: Change in resident's appearance

Hearing: Resident's words, tone, and breathing

Touch: Resident's skin and pulse

Fig. 2-2. Reporting what you observe means using more than one sense.

Sight. *Look for changes in appearance, including rashes, redness, paleness, swelling, discharge, weakness, sunken eyes, posture or gait (walking) changes.*

Hearing. *Listen to what the resident tells you about his condition, family, or needs. Is he speaking clearly and making sense? Does he show emotions, such as anger, frustration, or sadness? Is breathing normal? Does he wheeze, gasp, or cough? Is the area calm and quiet enough for him to rest as needed?*

Touch. *Does the skin feel hot or cool, moist or dry? Is pulse rate regular?*

Smell. *Do you notice odor from the resident's body? Odors could suggest inadequate bathing, infections, or incontinence.* **Incontinence** *is the inability to control the bladder or bowels. Breath odor could suggest use of alcohol or tobacco, indigestion, or poor oral care.*

Using all your senses will allow you to make the most complete report of a resident's situation.

Even for an oral report, write notes so you do not forget important details. Following an oral report, document when, why, about what, and to whom an oral report was given. Use your notes to write these reports. Do not rely on memory.

Sometimes the nurse or another member of the care team will give you a brief oral report on a resident. Listen carefully. Take notes if you need to (Fig. 2-3). Ask about anything you do not understand. At the end of the report, restate what you have been told to make sure you understand it.

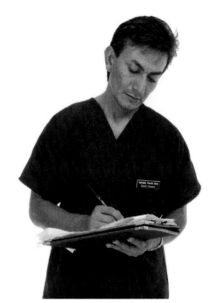

Fig. 2-3. Take notes on oral reports if you need to.

In your training, you will learn medical terms for specific conditions. Medical terms are made up of word parts. These parts are roots, prefixes, and suffixes. A root is the part of a word that gives it meaning. A prefix comes at the front of the word. It works with a word root to make a new term. A suffix is found at the end of a word. A suffix by itself does not form a full word. When you add a prefix or a root, the suffix turns it into a working medical term.

Here are some examples:

• The root "scope" means "an instrument to look inside." The prefix "oto" means "ear." An otoscope is an instrument used to examine the ear.

• The prefix "brady" means "slow." The root "cardia" means "heart." "Bradycardia" is slow heart rate or pulse.

• The suffix "meter" means "measuring instrument." The prefix "thermo" means "heat." A thermometer is an instrument that measures temperature.

2

Foundations of Resident Care

When speaking with residents and their families, use simple, non-medical terms. When you speak with the care team, medical terms will help you give more complete information.

Abbreviations are a way to communicate more efficiently. For example, the abbreviation "p.r.n." means "as necessary." Learn the standard medical abbreviations your facility uses. Use them to report information briefly and accurately. You may need to know these abbreviations to read assignments or care plans. **You will find a list of medical abbreviations at the end of this book.**

Telephone Communication

At times, you may answer the telephone at your facility. General rules for speaking on the phone are:

- Be cheerful when greeting a caller. Say, "Good morning," "Good afternoon," or "Good evening."

- Identify your facility: "Lincolnwood Facility."

- Identify yourself and your position: "Nancy Jones, Nursing Assistant."

- Listen closely to the caller's request. Write down messages. Ask for correct spelling of names.

- Get a telephone number, if needed.

- Say "Thank you," and "Goodbye."

Do not give out any information about staff or residents over the phone. All resident and staff information is confidential. It must not be given over the telephone. Refer this type of phone call to a supervisor. You may place a caller on hold if you need to get someone to take the call. Ask the caller if she can hold first.

Unit 2. **Describe barriers to communication**

Communication can be blocked or disrupted in many ways (Fig. 2-4). These are some barriers and ways to avoid them:

Resident does not hear you, does not hear correctly, or does not understand. Directly face the resident. Speak more slowly than you do with family and friends. Speak clearly. Use a low, pleasant voice. Do not whisper or mumble.

Resident is difficult to understand. Be patient. Take time to listen. Ask resident to repeat or explain. State the message in your own words to make sure you have under-

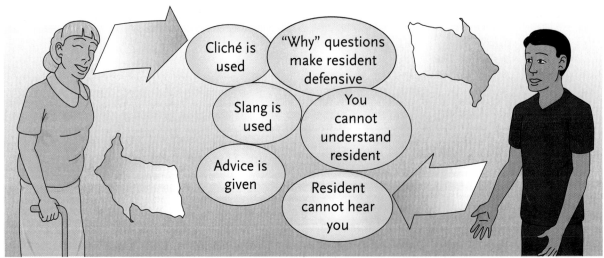

Fig. 2-4. **Barriers to communication.**

stood. Use a pen and paper or communication board (see chapter 8) to communicate.

Message uses words receiver does not understand. Do not use medical terms with residents. Speak in simple, everyday words. Ask what a word means if you are not sure.

Do not use slang words. Do not curse. Slang can confuse the message. Avoid slang; it is unprofessional and may not be understood. Do not curse or use profanity, even if the resident does.

Avoid clichés. Clichés are phrases that are used repeatedly and do not really mean anything. Instead, listen to what is really being said. Respond with a meaningful message.

Giving advice is inappropriate. Do not offer your opinion or advice. Giving medical advice is not within your scope of practice. It could be dangerous.

Asking "why" makes the resident defensive. Avoid asking "why" when a resident speaks. "Why" questions make people feel defensive.

Yes/no answers end a conversation. Ask open-ended questions. They require more than a "yes" or "no" answer.

Get to know your residents. Respect what they want to talk about.

Defense mechanisms may be considered barriers to communication. **Defense mechanisms** are unconscious behaviors used to release tension or cope with stress. They help to block uncomfortable or threatening feelings. They include the following:

- **Denial**: Rejecting the thought or feeling— "I'm not upset with you!"

- **Projection**: Seeing feelings in others that are really one's own—"My teacher hates me."

- **Displacement**: Transferring a strong negative feeling to a safer place. For example, an unhappy employee cannot yell at his boss for fear of losing his job. He later yells at his wife.

- **Rationalization**: Making excuses to justify a situation—After stealing something, saying, "Everybody does it."

- **Repression**: Blocking painful thoughts or feelings from the mind—For example, forgetting sexual abuse.

- **Regression**: Going back to an old, usually immature behavior—For example, throwing a temper tantrum as an adult.

Culture can affect communication. A **culture** is a system of behaviors people learn from the people they live and grow up with. Each person's background, values, and language affect how we communicate. When you communicate with residents from different cultures, ask yourself:

- What information do I need to communicate to this person?

- Does this person speak English as a first or second language?

- Do I speak this person's language, or do I need an interpreter?

- Does this person have any cultural practices about touch or gestures I should adapt to?

Unit 3. List guidelines for communicating with residents with special needs

Residents who have special needs require special communication techniques. Special techniques may be required for these conditions or illnesses:

- hearing or visual impairments
- mental illness
- combative or inappropriate behavior
- dementia

Information on communicating with residents who have had a stroke or who have Alzheimer's disease is in chapter 8.

Hearing Impairment

Persons who have impaired hearing or are deaf may have lost their hearing gradually, or they may have been born deaf. Use the following guidelines to make communication more effective.

Guidelines
Hearing Impairment

- If the person has a hearing aid, make sure he or she is wearing it and that it is working properly (Fig. 2-5). There are many types of hearing aids. Follow manufacturer's directions for cleaning. In general, the hearing aid needs to be cleaned daily. Wipe it with alcohol using a tissue or soft cloth. Do not put it in water. Handle the hearing aid carefully. Do not drop it. Always store it inside its case when it is not worn. Turn it off when it is not in use. Remove it before showers or when bathing resident and during the night. When storing it for an extended period of time, remove the battery.

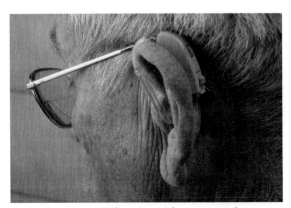

Fig. 2-5. **Make sure hearing aids are turned on.**

- Reduce or remove background noise, such as TVs, radios, and loud speech. Close doors if you have to.
- Get residents' attention before speaking. Do not startle them by approaching from behind. Walk in front or touch them lightly on the arm to show you are near.
- Speak clearly, slowly, and in good lighting. Directly face the person (Fig. 2-6). The light should be on your face, not on the resident's. Ask if he can hear what you are saying.
- Do not shout. Do not mouth the words in an exaggerated way.

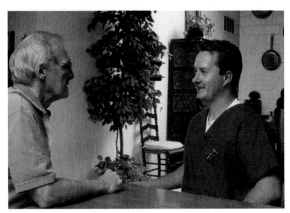

Fig. 2-6. **Speak face-to-face in good light.**

- Lower the pitch of your voice.
- Do not chew gum or eat while speaking. Keep your hands away from your face while talking.
- Know which ear hears better. Try to speak to that side.
- Use short sentences and simple words.
- Repeat what you have said using different words, when needed. Some hearing-impaired people want you to repeat exactly what was said. This is because they miss only a few words.
- Use picture cards or a notepad as needed.
- Hearing decline can be a normal aspect of aging. Be matter-of-fact about this. Be understanding and supportive.

Vision Impairment

Vision impairment can affect people of all ages. It can exist at birth or develop gradually. It can occur in one eye or both. It can also be the result of injury, illness, or aging.

Guidelines
Vision Impairment

- If the person has glasses, make sure they are clean and that he or she wears them. Clean glass lenses with water and soft tissue. Clean plastic lenses with cleaning fluid and a lens cloth. Also, make sure that glasses are in good condition and fit well. If they do not, tell the nurse.

- Knock on the door and identify yourself when you enter the room. Do not touch the resident until you have said your name. Explain what you would like to do. Tell the resident when you are leaving.

- Always tell the resident what you are doing while caring for him. Give specific directions, such as, "On your right" or, "In front of you."

- Provide good lighting at all times. Face the resident when speaking.

- When you enter a new room with the resident, orient him or her to the area. Describe the things you see around you. Do not use words such as "see," "look," and "watch."

- Tell the resident where the call light is.

- Use the face of an imaginary clock as a guide to explain the position of objects that are in front of resident (Fig. 2-7).

- Do not move personal items or furniture without the resident's permission.

- Leave the door completely open or completely closed.

- Offer large-print newspapers, magazines, and books.

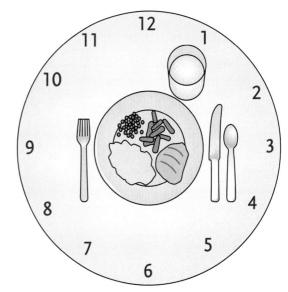

Fig. 2-7. The face of a clock can explain the position of objects.

- Encourage the use of the other senses, such as hearing, touch, and smell. Encourage the resident to feel and touch things, such as clothing, furniture, or items in the room.

- Use large clocks, clocks that chime, and radios to help keep track of time.

- Get books on tape and other aids from the library or support organizations.

Mental Illness

Mental health is the normal function of emotional and intellectual abilities. Characteristics of a person who is mentally healthy include the ability to:

- get along with others (Fig. 2-8)

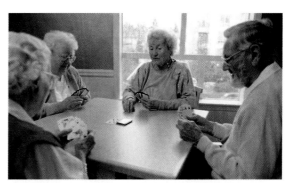

Fig. 2-8. The ability to interact well with other people is a characteristic of mental health.

- adapt to change

- care for self and others

- give and accept love

- deal with situations that cause stress, disappointment, and frustration

- take responsibility for decisions, feelings, and actions

- control and fulfill desires and impulses appropriately

Although it involves the emotions and mental functions, mental illness is a disease. It is like any physical disease. It produces signs and symptoms. It affects the body's ability to function. It responds to proper treatment and care. Mental illness disrupts a person's ability to function at a normal level in the family, home, or community. It often causes inappropriate behavior. Different types of mental illness will affect how well residents communicate.

Mentally healthy people are able to control their emotions and actions. Mentally ill people may not have this control. Mentally ill people cannot simply choose to be well. Knowing that mental illness is a disease much like any physical illness helps you work with mentally ill residents.

Guidelines
Mental Illness

- Do not talk to adults as if they were children.

- Use simple, clear statements. Use a normal tone of voice.

- Be sure that what you say and how you speak show respect and concern.

- Sit or stand at a normal distance from the resident. Be aware of your body language.

- Be honest and direct, as with any resident.

- Avoid arguments.

- Maintain eye contact.

- Listen carefully (Fig. 2-9).

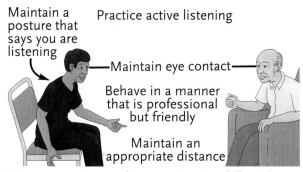

Fig. 2-9. Practice good communication skills with mentally ill residents.

See unit 10 in chapter 8 for more information on mental illness.

Combative Behavior

Residents may display **combative**, meaning violent or hostile, behavior. Such behavior includes hitting, pushing, kicking, or verbal attacks. It may result from disease affecting the brain. It may also be due to frustration. It may just be part of someone's personality. In general, combative behavior is not a reaction to you. Try not to take it personally.

Always report and document combative behavior. Even if you are not upset, the care team needs to be aware of it.

Guidelines
Combative Behavior

- Remain calm.

- Block physical blows or step out of the way, but never hit back (Fig. 2-10).

- Leave the resident alone if you can safely do so.

- Do not respond to verbal attacks.

- Consider what provoked the resident.

- Report inappropriate behavior to the nurse.

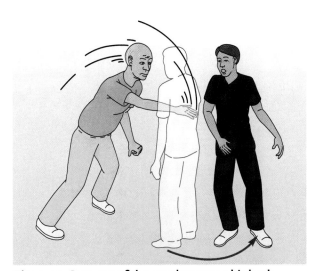

Fig. 2-10. Step out of the way but never hit back.

Anger

Anger is a natural emotion. Residents and their families may express it. There are many causes of anger. Some are disease, fear, pain, loneliness, and loss of independence. Anger may just be a part of someone's personality. Anger is expressed in different ways. Some are shouting, yelling, threatening, throwing things, and pacing. Others express anger by withdrawing, being silent, or sulking. Always report angry behavior to the nurse.

Guidelines
Angry Behavior

- Stay calm.

- Do not respond to verbal attacks. Do not argue.

- Empathize with the resident. Try to understand what he or she is feeling.

- Try to find out what caused the resident's anger. Using silence may help the resident explain. Listen attentively as the resident speaks.

- Treat the resident with dignity and respect. Explain what you are going to do and when you will do it.

- Answer call lights promptly.

- Stay at a safe distance if the resident becomes combative.

Inappropriate Behavior

Some residents will show inappropriate behavior. This includes sexual advances and comments. Sexual advances include any sexual words, comments, or behavior that makes you feel uncomfortable. Report this behavior to the nurse immediately.

Inappropriate behavior also includes residents removing their clothes or touching themselves in public. Illness, dementia, confusion, and medication may cause this behavior. If you encounter any embarrassing situation, be matter-of-fact. Do not overreact. This may actually reinforce the behavior. Try to distract the person. If that does not work, gently direct the resident to a private area. Notify the nurse.

Confused residents may have problems that mimic inappropriate sexual behavior. They may have an uncomfortable rash; clothes that are too tight, too hot, or too scratchy; or the need to go to the bathroom. Consider and watch for these problems. When residents act inappropriately, report it, even if you think it was harmless.

Unit 4. Identify ways to promote safety and handle non-medical emergencies

Safety

Prevention is the key to safety. Report unsafe conditions to your supervisor *before* accidents occur. As you work, watch for safety hazards. Before leaving a resident's room, look around and do a final check. Ask yourself:

- Is the call light within reach?

- Is the room tidy? Are the resident's items in their proper places?
- Are the side rails up if they are ordered?
- Is the furniture in the same place as you found it? Is the bed in its lowest position?
- Does the resident have a clear walkway around the room and into the bathroom?

📄 *Staff have the responsibility to keep the resident safe from harm. The state agency survey team will look for safety hazards in the environment.*

Principles of Body Mechanics

Body mechanics is the way the parts of the body work together when you move. Good body mechanics help save energy and prevent injury.

The ABC's of good body mechanics are:

- **Alignment.** When standing, sitting, or lying down, try to have your body in alignment. This means that the two sides of the body are mirror images of each other. Maintain correct body alignment when lifting or carrying an object by keeping it close to your body. Point your feet and body in the direction you are moving. Avoid twisting at the waist (Fig. 2-11).
- **Base of support.** The base of support is the foundation of an object. The feet are the body's base of support. Standing with your legs shoulder-width apart gives a greater base of support. You will be more stable than someone standing with his or her feet close together.
- **Center of gravity.** The center of gravity in your body is the point where the most weight is concentrated. This point will depend on the position of the body. When you stand, your weight is centered in your pelvis. A low center of gravity gives a more stable base of support.

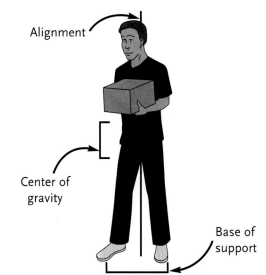

Fig. 2-11. Proper body alignment is important when standing and when sitting.

Some examples of using good body mechanics include:

- **Lifting a heavy object from the floor.** Spread your feet shoulder-width apart. Bend your knees. Using the strong, large muscles in your thighs, upper arms, and shoulders, lift the object. Pull it close to your body, level with your pelvis. By doing this, you keep the object close to your center of gravity and base of support. When you stand up, push with your strong hip and thigh muscles. Raise your body and the object together (Fig. 2-12).

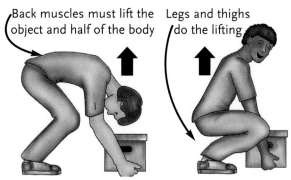

Fig. 2-12. In this illustration, which person is lifting correctly?

- **Do not twist when you are moving an object.** Always face the object or person you are moving. Pivot your feet instead of twisting at the waist.

- **Helping a resident sit up, stand up, or walk.** Whenever you support a resident's weight, assume a good stance. Place your feet 12 inches, or hip-width, apart. Put one foot in front of the other, with your knees bent. Your upper body should stay upright and in alignment.

- **Bend your knees to lower yourself, rather than bending from the waist.** When a task requires bending, use a good stance. This lets you use the big muscles in your legs and hips rather than the smaller muscles in your back.

- **If you are making a bed, adjust the height to a safe working level, usually waist high.** Avoid bending at the waist.

Keep the following tips in mind to avoid strain and injury:

- Assess the situation first. Clear the path. Remove any obstacles.

- Get help when possible for lifting or helping residents.

- Use both arms and hands to lift, pull, push, or carry objects.

- Hold objects close to you when you are lifting or carrying them (Fig. 2-13).

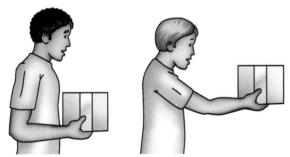

Fig. 2-13. Holding things close to you moves weight toward your center of gravity. In this illustration, who is more likely to strain his back muscles?

- Push, slide, or pull objects rather than lifting them.

- Avoid bending and reaching as much as possible. Move or position furniture so that you do not have to bend or reach.

- When moving a resident, let him know what you will do so he can help if possible. Count to three. Lift or move on three so everyone moves together.

- Report to the nurse any task that you feel you cannot safely do. Never try to lift an object or a resident that you feel you cannot handle.

Accident Prevention

Falls

Most accidents in a facility are falls. Falls can be caused by an unsafe environment or by loss of abilities. Falls are particularly common among the elderly. Older people are often more seriously injured by falls, as their bones are more fragile.

Factors that raise the risk of falls include:

- clutter

- throw rugs

- exposed electrical cords

- slippery or wet floors

- uneven floors or stairs

- poor lighting

- call lights that are out of reach or not promptly answered

Personal conditions that raise the risk of falls include medications, loss of vision, gait or balance problems, weakness, paralysis, and disorientation. **Disorientation** means confusion about person, place or time.

To guard against falls:

- Clear all walkways of clutter, throw rugs, and cords.

- Use non-skid mats or carpeting where needed. Have residents wear non-skid shoes. Make sure shoelaces are tied.

- Have residents wear clothing that fits properly, e.g. that is not too long.

- Keep frequently-used items close to residents, including call lights. Answer call lights promptly.

- If ordered, check placement of body or bed alarms and to see if they are working.

- Immediately clean up spills.

- Report loose hand rails immediately.

- Mark uneven flooring or stairs with colored tape to indicate a hazard.

- Improve lighting where needed.

- Lock wheelchairs before helping residents into or out of them. Lock bed wheels before helping a resident into and out of bed or when giving care.

- Return beds to their lowest position when you have finished with care. Place floor mats as ordered.

- Monitor bed or body alarms if used.

- Get help when moving residents. Do not assume you can do it alone.

- Offer trips to the bathroom often. Respond to requests promptly.

- Leave furniture in the same place.

- Know residents who are at risk for falls and provide help.

If a resident starts to fall, be in a good position to help support him or her. Never try to catch a falling resident. Rather, use your body to slide him or her to the floor. If you try to reverse a fall, you may hurt yourself and/or the resident.

Burns/Scalds

Burns can be caused by stoves and appliances, hot water or liquids, or heating devices. Small children, older adults, or people with loss of sensation due to paralysis are at greatest risk of burns. **Scalds** are burns caused by hot liquids. Follow these guidelines to guard against burns and scalds:

- Always check water temperature with water thermometer or on wrist before using.

- Report frayed electrical cords or unsafe-looking appliances immediately. Do not use them. Remove them from the room.

- Let residents know you are about to pour or set down a hot liquid. Make sure residents are sitting down before serving hot drinks.

- Pour hot drinks away from residents.

- Keep hot drinks and liquids away from edges of tables. Put a lid on them.

- If plate warmers are used, monitor them carefully.

Poisoning

Facilities have many harmful substances that should not be swallowed. These include cleaners, paints, medicines, toiletries, and glues. These products should be stored or locked away from confused residents or those with limited vision. Do not leave cleaning products in residents' rooms. The number for the Poison Control Center should be posted by all telephones.

Poisonous chemicals must be kept in locked rooms or cabinets.

Choking

Choking can occur when eating, drinking or taking medication. People who are weak, ill, or unconscious may choke on their own saliva. To guard against choking, residents should eat sitting as upright as possible. Residents with swallowing problems may have a special diet with liquids thickened to the consistency of honey or syrup. Thickened liquids are easier to swallow. You will learn more about this in chapter 7.

Resident Identification

Residents must always be identified. Not

identifying residents before giving care or serving food can cause serious problems, even death. Facilities have different methods of identification. Some have ID bracelets. Some have pictures to identify residents. Identify each resident before starting any procedure or giving any care. Always identify residents before placing meal trays or helping with feeding. Check the diet card against the resident's identification. Call the resident by name.

Material Safety Data Sheet (MSDS)
The Occupational Safety and Health Administration (OSHA) is responsible for the safety of employees at work. OSHA requires that all dangerous chemicals have a Material Safety Data Sheet (MSDS). This sheet details the chemical ingredients, chemical dangers, emergency response actions to be taken, and safe handling procedures for the product. Some facilities use a toll-free number to access MSDS information. MSDSs must be accessible in work areas for all employees. Important information about the MSDS includes:

- Your employer must have a MSDS for every chemical used.

- Your employer must provide easy access to the MSDS.

- You must know where your MSDSs are kept and how to read them. If you do not know how, ask for help.

Fire
Most facilities have a fire safety plan. All workers need to be familiar with it. Fire and disaster drills help you learn what to do in an emergency. The nurse will explain your facility's guidelines. Remember to get the residents to safety first. A fast, calm and confident response by the staff saves lives.

Follow these guidelines to guard against fire:

- Never leave smokers unattended. If residents smoke, make sure they are in the proper area for smoking. Be sure that cigarettes are extinguished. Empty ashtrays often. Before emptying ashtrays, make sure there are no hot ashes or hot matches in ashtray.

- Report frayed or damaged electrical cords immediately. Report electrical equipment in need of repair immediately.

- Fire alarms and exit doors should not be blocked. If they are, report this to the nurse.

- Every facility will have a fire extinguisher (Fig. 2-14). The PASS acronym will help you understand how to use it:

Pull the pin.

Aim at the base of fire when spraying.

Squeeze the handle.

Sweep back and forth at the base of the fire.

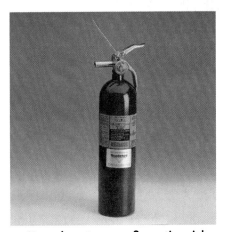

Fig. 2-14. Know how to use a fire extinguisher.

In case of fire, the RACE acronym is a good rule to follow:

- **R**emove residents from danger.
- **A**ctivate 911.
- **C**ontain fire if possible.
- **E**xtinguish, or fire department will extinguish.

Follow these guidelines for helping residents exit the building safely:

- Know the facility's fire evacuation plan.

- Know which residents require one-on-one assistance or assistive devices.

- Stay calm.

- Remove anything blocking a window or door that could be used as a fire exit.

- If clothing catches fire, do not run. Stop, drop to the ground, and roll to extinguish flames.

- Stay low in a room to escape a fire.

- Use a covering over the face to reduce smoke inhalation.

- Do not get into an elevator during a fire.

- Call for emergency help.

Disaster Guidelines

Nursing assistants need to be skilled and responsible during a disaster. An emergency or disaster may occur during working hours. Disasters can include fire, flood, earthquake, hurricane, tornado, or severe weather. Today, many facilities also consider acts of terrorism as disasters.

Annual in-services and disaster drills are held at facilities. Take advantage of these sessions. Pay close attention to instructions.

During an emergency, a nurse or the administrator will give directions. Listen carefully to all directions. Follow instructions. Know the locations of all exits and stairways. Know where the fire alarms and extinguishers are located.

Know the appropriate action to take in any situation. This protects you and your residents. Each facility has a disaster plan available for employees to learn. Make sure you know your facility's plan. Your instructor will have specific guidelines for disasters that commonly occur in your area.

The facility must have a plan to deal with disasters. The state agency survey team will evaluate staff participation in disaster training and drills.

Unit 5. Demonstrate how to recognize and respond to medical emergencies

Medical emergencies may be the result of accidents or sudden illnesses. This section discusses what to do in a medical emergency. Heart attacks, stroke, diabetic emergencies, choking, automobile accidents, and gunshot wounds are all medical emergencies. Falls, burns, and cuts can also be emergencies.

In an emergency, try to remain calm, act quickly, and communicate clearly. Knowing these steps will help:

- **Assess the situation**. Try to find out what has happened. Make sure you are not in danger. Notice the time.

- **Assess the victim**. Ask the injured or ill person what has happened. If the person cannot respond, he may be unconscious. Determine whether the person is conscious. Tap the person and ask if he is all right. Speak loudly. Use the person's name if you know it. If there is no response, assume that the person is unconscious. This is an emergency. *Call for help right away, or send someone else to call.*

If a person is conscious and able to speak, then he is breathing and has a pulse. Talk with the person about what happened. Check the person for injury. Look for these things:

- severe bleeding

- changes in consciousness
- irregular breathing
- unusual color or feel to the skin
- swollen places on the body
- medical alert tags
- anything the resident says is painful

If any of these exist, you may need professional medical help. Always get help before doing anything else.

If the injured or ill person is conscious, he may be frightened. Listen to the person. Tell him what is being done to help him. Be calm and confident. Reassure him that he is being taken care of.

After the emergency, you will need to document it in your notes. Only report the facts. Complete an incident report. An **incident** is an accident or an unexpected event during the course of care. It is not part of the normal routine in a facility. State and federal guidelines require incidents to be recorded in an incident report. Report an incident to the nurse as soon as possible. The information in an incident report is confidential.

First aid is care given in an emergency before trained medical professionals can take over. **Cardiopulmonary resuscitation** (**CPR**) refers to medical procedures used when a person's heart or lungs have stopped working. CPR is used until medical help arrives.

Quick action is necessary. CPR must be started immediately. Brain damage may occur within 4–6 minutes after the heart stops beating and the lungs stop breathing. The person can die within 10 minutes.

Only properly trained people should perform CPR. Your employer will probably arrange for you to be trained in CPR. If not, ask about American Heart Association or Red Cross CPR training. CPR is an important skill to learn. If you are not trained, do not attempt to perform CPR.

Know your facility's policies on whether you can initiate CPR if you have been trained. Some facilities do not allow NAs to begin CPR without direction of the nurse.

This textbook is not a CPR course. The following is a brief review for people who have had CPR training. It is a procedure to use on adults, not children.

1. Check to see if the person is responsive. Gently shake the person and shout, "Are you okay?"

2. If there is no response, call 911 immediately or send someone to call 911. Stay calm.

3. Kneel at the person's side near his head to start CPR.

4. Open the airway. Tilt the head back slightly. Lift the chin with one hand while pushing down on the forehead with the other hand (head tilt-chin lift method) (Fig. 2-15). This method is used if a neck injury is not suspected.

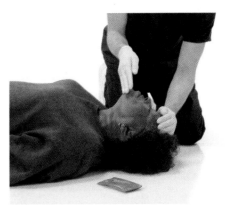

Fig. 2-15. The head tilt-chin lift method.

5. Hold the airway open and check for breathing:
   - Look for the chest to rise and fall.

- Listen for sounds of breathing. Put your ear near the person's nose and mouth.

- Feel for the person's breath on your cheek.

6. If the person is still not breathing, you will have to breathe for the person. Give two rescue breaths. To give rescue breaths:

- Pinch the nose to keep air from escaping. Cover the person's mouth completely with your mouth.

- If a barrier device, such as a special face mask, is available, use it to give rescue breaths (Fig. 2-16).

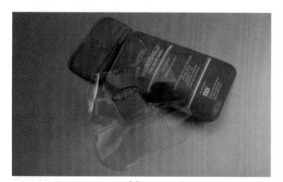

Fig. 2-16. One type of face mask.

- Blow into the person's mouth slowly. Watch for the chest to rise (Fig. 2-17). Blow two full breaths, about two seconds each. Turn your head to the side to listen for air. If the chest does not rise when you give a rescue breath, reopen the airway. Use the head tilt-chin lift method. Try to give rescue breaths again.

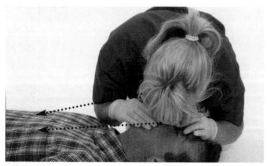

Fig. 2-17.

7. After giving rescue breaths, look for signs of response. The person may start moving, breathing normally, or coughing. If you do not see a response, give 30 chest compressions. Do this only if you have been trained to do so. Be sure the person is lying flat on a hard surface. To give chest compressions:

- Place your hands in the center of the person's chest between the nipples. Place one hand on top of the other. Interlace your fingers to help maintain hand position.

- Place knees shoulder-width apart and as close to the person as possible. Bring your body up and forward. Your shoulders should be directly above your hands. Lock your elbows and shoulders.

- Press the heel of your hand into the chest. Do not allow hands to lose contact with the chest during compressions.

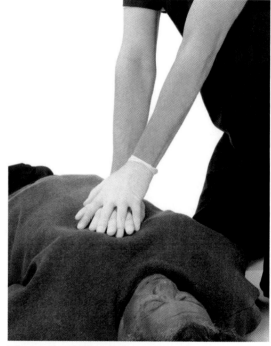

Fig. 2-18. Giving chest compressions.

- Use the heel of your hand to give 30 chest compressions. After about a minute of CPR, check for signs of response. If you see signs of response, stop compressions. Continue to provide rescue breathing as necessary (one breath every five seconds).

When medical help arrives, follow their directions. Assist them as necessary.

Choking

When something is blocking the tube through which air enters the lungs, the person has an **obstructed airway**. When people are choking, they usually put their hands to their throats and cough (Fig. 2-19). As long as the person can speak, cough, or breathe, do nothing. Encourage her to cough as forcefully as possible to get the object out. Ask someone to get a nurse. Stay with the person until she stops choking or can no longer speak, cough, or breathe. Do not hit her on the back.

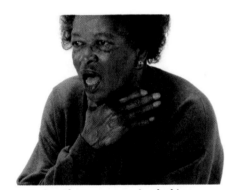

Fig. 2-19. A sign that a person is choking.

If a person can no longer speak, cough, or breathe, or turns blue, call for help immediately. Time is of extreme importance. Abdominal thrusts are a method of attempting to remove an object from the airway of someone who is choking. These thrusts work to remove the blockage upward, out of the throat. Make sure the person needs help before giving abdominal thrusts. If the person cannot speak, cough, or breathe, or if her response is weak, give abdominal thrusts. Do this only if your facility allows it.

Abdominal thrusts for the conscious person

1. **Stand behind the person. Bring your arms under her arms. Wrap your arms around the person's waist.**

2. **Make a fist with one hand. Place the flat, thumb side of the fist against the person's abdomen, above the navel but below the breastbone.**

3. **Grasp the fist with your other hand. Pull both hands toward you and up (inward and upward), quickly and forcefully (Fig. 2-20).**

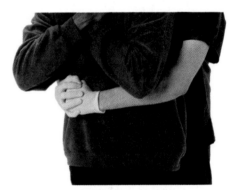

Fig. 2-20.

4. **Repeat until the object is pushed out or the person loses consciousness.**

Do not practice this procedure on a live person. This risks injury to the ribs or internal organs. If the person becomes unconscious while choking, help her to the floor gently. Lie her on her back with her face up. Make sure help is on the way. She may have a completely blocked airway. She needs professional medical help immediately.

Shock

Shock occurs when organs and tissues in the body do not receive an adequate blood supply. Bleeding, heart attack, severe infection, and falling blood pressure can lead to shock. Shock can become worse when the person is frightened or in severe pain.

Shock is a dangerous, life-threatening situation. Signs of shock include pale or bluish skin, staring, increased pulse and respiration rates, low blood pressure, and extreme thirst. Always call for help if you suspect a person is in shock. To prevent or treat shock, do the following:

Shock

1.   **Have the person lie down on her back. If the person is bleeding from the mouth or vomiting, place her on her side (unless you suspect that the neck, back, or spinal cord is injured).**

2.   **Control bleeding. This procedure is described later in the chapter.**

3.   **Check pulse and respirations if possible. (See chapter 6.)**

4.   **Keep the person as calm and comfortable as possible.**

5.   **Maintain normal body temperature. If the weather is cold, place a blanket around the person. If the weather is hot, provide shade.**

6.   **Elevate the feet unless the person has a head or abdominal injury, breathing difficulties, or a fractured bone or back (Fig. 2-21). Elevate the head and shoulders if a head wound or breathing difficulties are present. Never elevate a body part if a broken bone exists.**

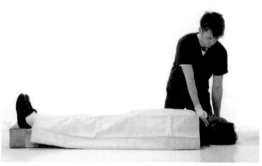

Fig. 2-21.

7.   **Do not give the person anything to eat or drink.**

8.   **Call for help immediately. Victims of shock should always receive medical care as soon as possible.**

Insulin Shock and Diabetic Coma

Insulin shock and diabetic coma are problems of diabetes that can be life-threatening. Insulin shock can result from either too much insulin or too little food. It occurs when insulin is given and the person skips a meal or does not eat all the food required. Even when a regular amount of food is eaten, physical activity may rapidly absorb the food. This causes too much insulin to be in the body. Vomiting and diarrhea may also lead to insulin shock in people with diabetes.

The first signs of insulin shock include feeling weak or different, nervousness, dizziness, and perspiration. These signal that the resident needs food in a form that can be rapidly absorbed. Call the nurse if the resident has shown signs of insulin shock. Signs and symptoms of insulin shock include:

*   hunger
*   weakness
*   rapid pulse
*   headache
*   low blood pressure
*   perspiration
*   cold, clammy skin
*   confusion
*   trembling
*   nervousness
*   blurred vision
*   numbness of the lips and tongue
*   unconsciousness

Having too little insulin causes diabetic coma. It can result from undiagnosed dia-

2

Foundations of Resident Care

betes, not enough insulin, eating too much, not getting enough exercise, and physical or emotional stress.

The signs of onset of diabetic coma include increased thirst or urination, abdominal pain, deep or difficult breathing, and breath that smells sweet or fruity. Call the nurse immediately if you think your resident is experiencing diabetic coma. Other signs and symptoms of diabetic coma include:

- hunger
- weakness
- rapid, weak pulse
- headache
- low blood pressure
- dry skin
- flushed cheeks
- drowsiness
- slow, deep, and labored breathing
- nausea and vomiting
- abdominal pain
- sweet, fruity breath odor
- air hunger, or resident gasping for air and being unable to catch his breath
- unconsciousness

See chapter 8 for more information on diabetes and related care.

CVA or Stroke
The medical term for a stroke is a cerebrovascular accident (CVA). CVA, or stroke, is caused when a clot or a ruptured blood vessel suddenly cuts off blood supply to the brain. Symptoms that a stroke is beginning include dizziness, ringing in the ears, blurred vision, headache, nausea, vomiting, slurring of words, and loss of memory. These signs and symptoms should be reported immediately.

A transient ischemic attack, or TIA, is a warning sign of a stroke. It is the result of a temporary lack of oxygen in the brain. Symptoms may last up to 24 hours. They include tingling, weakness, or some loss of movement in an arm or leg. These symptoms should not be ignored. Report them to the nurse immediately. Signs that a stroke is occurring include:

- loss of consciousness
- redness in the face
- noisy breathing
- dizziness
- blurred vision
- ringing in the ears
- headache
- nausea/vomiting
- seizures
- loss of bowel and bladder control
- paralysis on one side of the body
- weakness on one side of the body
- the inability to speak or to speak clearly
- facial droop
- use of strange words
- elevated blood pressure
- slow pulse rate

See chapter 8 for more information.

Myocardial Infarction or Heart Attack
When blood flow to the heart is completely blocked, oxygen and nutrients fail to reach its cells. Waste products are not removed. The muscle cell dies. This is called a myocardial infarction (MI), or heart attack. The area of dead tissue may be large or small. This depends on the artery involved.

A myocardial infarction is an emergency that can result in serious heart damage or death. The following are signs and symptoms of MI:

- sudden, severe pain in the chest, usually on the left side or in the center, behind the breastbone
- pain or discomfort in other areas of the body, such as one or both arms, the back, neck, jaw, or stomach
- indigestion or heartburn
- nausea and vomiting
- dyspnea, or difficulty breathing
- dizziness
- pale, gray, or bluish (cyanotic) skin color, indicating lack of oxygen
- perspiration
- cold and clammy skin
- weak and irregular pulse rate
- low blood pressure
- anxiety and a sense of doom
- denial of a heart problem

The pain of a heart attack is commonly described as a crushing, pressing, squeezing, stabbing, piercing pain, or, "like someone is sitting on my chest." The pain may go down the inside of the left arm. A person may also feel it in the neck and/or in the jaw. The pain usually does not go away.

As with men, women's most common symptom is chest pain or discomfort. But women are somewhat more likely than men to have shortness of breath, nausea/vomiting, and back or jaw pain.

You must take immediate action if a resident has any of these symptoms. Follow these steps:

Heart attack

1.   **Call or have someone call the nurse.**

2.   **Place the person in a comfortable position. Encourage him to rest. Reassure him that you will not leave him alone.**

3.   **Loosen the clothing around the person's neck (Fig. 2-22).**

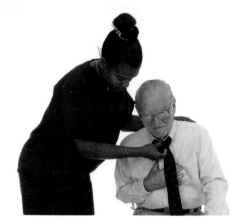

Fig. 2-22.

4.   **Do not give the person liquids or food.**

5.   **Monitor the person's breathing and pulse. If the person stops breathing or has no pulse, perform rescue breathing or CPR only if you are trained to do so and if your facility allows it.**

6.   **Stay with the person until help arrives.**

See chapter 8 for more information on heart attacks.

Fainting

Fainting occurs as a result of decreased blood flow to the brain, causing a loss of consciousness. Fainting may be the result of hunger, fear, pain, fatigue, standing for a long time, poor ventilation, or overheating. Signs and symptoms of fainting include dizziness, perspiration, pale skin, weak pulse, shallow respirations, and blackness in the visual field. If someone appears likely to faint, follow these steps:

Fainting

1.   **Have the person lie down or sit down before fainting occurs.**

2. If the person is in a sitting position, have her bend forward and place her head between her knees (Fig. 2-23). If the person is lying flat on her back, elevate the legs.

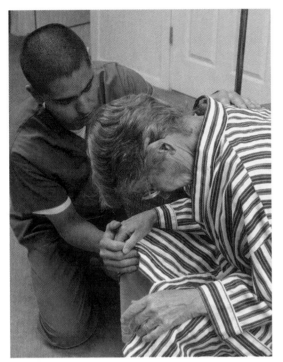

Fig. 2-23.

3. Loosen any tight clothing.

4. Have the person stay in position for at least five minutes after symptoms disappear.

5. Help the person get up slowly. Continue to observe her for symptoms of fainting. Stay with her until she feels better. If you need help but cannot leave the person, use the call light.

6. Report the incident to the nurse.

If a person does faint, lower her to the floor or other flat surface. Position her on her back. Elevate her legs 8 to 12 inches. Loosen any tight clothing. Check to make sure the person is breathing. She should recover quickly, but keep her lying down for several minutes. Report the incident to the nurse immediately. Fainting may be a sign of a more serious medical condition.

Seizures

Seizures are involuntary, often violent, contractions of muscles. They can involve a small area or the entire body. Seizures are caused by an abnormality in the brain. They can occur in young children who have a high fever. Older children and adults who have a serious illness, fever, head injury, or epilepsy may also have seizures.

The main goal of a caregiver during a seizure is to make sure the resident is safe. During a seizure, a person may shake severely and thrust arms and legs uncontrollably. He may clench his jaw, drool, and be unable to swallow. Take the following emergency measures if a resident has a seizure:

Seizures

1. Lower the person to the floor. Lay him on his side.

2. Have someone call the nurse immediately. Do not leave the person unless you must do so to get medical help.

3. Move furniture away to prevent injury. If a pillow is nearby, place it under his head.

4. Do not try to restrain the person.

5. Do not force anything between the person's teeth. Do not place your hands in his mouth for any reason. You could be bitten.

6. Do not give liquids or food.

7. When the seizure is over, check breathing.

8. Report the length of the seizure and your observations to the nurse.

Bleeding

Severe bleeding can cause death quickly. It must be controlled. Call the nurse immediately. Then follow these steps to control bleeding:

Bleeding

1. Put on gloves. Take time to do this. If the resident is able, he can hold his bare hand over the wound until you can put on gloves.

2. Hold a thick sterile pad, a clean pad, or a clean cloth, handkerchief, or towel against the wound.

3. Press down hard directly on the bleeding wound until help arrives. Do not decrease pressure (Fig. 2-24). Put additional pads over the first pad if blood seeps through. Do not remove the first pad.

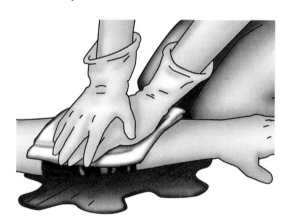

Fig. 2-24

4. If you can, raise the wound above the level of the heart to slow down the bleeding. If the wound is on an arm, leg, hand, or foot, and there are no broken bones, prop up the limb on towels, blankets, coats, or other absorbent material.

5. When bleeding is under control, secure the dressing to keep it in place. Check the person for symptoms of shock (pale skin, increased pulse and respiration rates, low blood pressure, and extreme thirst). Stay with the person until help arrives.

6. Remove gloves and wash hands thoroughly when finished.

Unit 6. Describe and demonstrate infection control practices

Infection control is the set of methods used to control and prevent the spread of disease. It is the responsibility of all members of the care team. Know your facility's infection control policies and procedures. They help protect you, residents, and others from disease.

A **microorganism** is a tiny living thing. It is not visible to the eye without a microscope. Microorganisms are always present in the environment. Infections occur when harmful microorganisms, called **pathogens**, enter the body. For infections to develop, pathogens must invade and grow within the human body. **Asepsis** means no pathogens are present. It refers to the clean conditions you want to create in your facility. In health care, an object can only be called "clean" if it has not been contaminated with pathogens. An object that is "dirty" has been contaminated with pathogens.

There are two main types of infections, systemic and localized. A **systemic infection** occurs when pathogens enter the bloodstream and move throughout the body. It causes general symptoms such as fever, chills, or mental confusion. A **localized infection** is limited to a specific part of the body. It has local symptoms. Its symptoms are near the site of infection. For example, if a wound becomes infected, the area around it may become red, hot, and painful. Another type of infection is a nosocomial infection. A **nosocomial infection**, or hospital-acquired infection (HAI), is an infection acquired in a hospital or other healthcare facility.

Preventing the spread of infection is important. To understand how to prevent disease you must first know how it is spread. The **chain of infection** describes how disease is transmitted from one being to another (Fig. 2-25). Definitions and examples of the six links in the chain of infection are:

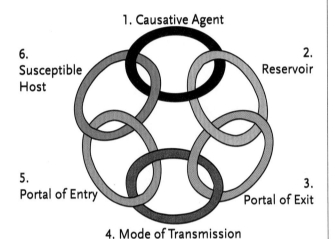

Fig. 2-25. The chain of infection.

Link 1: The **causative agent** is a pathogen or microorganism that causes disease. Normal flora are the microorganisms that live in and on the body. They do not cause harm. When they enter a different part of the body, they may cause an infection. Causative agents include bacteria, viruses, fungi, and protozoa.

Link 2: A **reservoir** is where the pathogen lives and grows. It can be a person, animal, plant, soil, or substance. Microorganisms grow best in warm, dark, and moist places where food is present. Reservoirs include the lungs, blood, and large intestine.

Link 3: The **portal of exit** is any body opening on an infected person allowing pathogens to leave. These include the nose, mouth, eyes, or a cut in skin (Fig. 2-26).

Link 4: The **mode of transmission** describes how the pathogen travels from one person to another. Transmission can happen through the air. It can also occur through direct or indirect contact. Direct contact happens by touching the infected person or his

or her secretions. Indirect contact results from touching something contaminated by the infected person, such as a tissue or clothes.

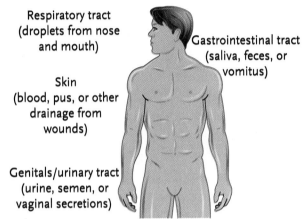

Fig. 2-26. Portals of exit.

Link 5: The **portal of entry** is any body opening on an uninfected person that allows pathogens to enter. This includes the nose, the mouth, the eyes, other mucous membranes, a cut in the skin, or dry/cracked skin (Fig. 2-27).

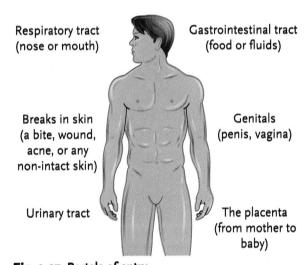

Fig. 2-27. Portals of entry.

Link 6: A **susceptible host** is an uninfected person who could get sick. This includes all healthcare workers and anyone in their care who is not already infected.

If one of the links in the chain of infection is broken, then the spread of infection stops.

Infection control practices help stop pathogens from traveling (Link 4), and getting on your hands, nose, eyes, mouth, skin, etc. (Link 5). You can also reduce your own chances of getting sick (Link 6) by having immunizations for diseases such as hepatitis B and influenza.

Standard Precautions and Transmission-Based Precautions

State and federal government agencies have guidelines and laws concerning infection control. The **Centers for Disease Control and Prevention** (**CDC**) is a federal agency that issues guidelines to protect and improve health. The CDC tries to control and prevent disease. In 1996, the CDC recommended a new infection control system to reduce the risk of contracting infectious diseases. In 2004, the CDC proposed some changes to this system. There are two levels of precautions within the infection control system. They are Standard Precautions and Transmission-Based, or Isolation, Precautions. In the 2004 proposed guidelines the CDC suggests that the term "Expanded Precautions" be used instead of "Transmission-Based Precautions."

Following Standard Precautions means treating all blood, body fluids, non-intact skin (like abrasions, pimples, or open sores), and mucous membranes (lining of mouth, nose, eyes, rectum, or genitals) as if they were infected. This is the only safe way of doing your job. You cannot tell by looking at your residents or their charts if they have a contagious disease such as HIV, hepatitis, or influenza.

Under Standard Precautions, "body fluids" include saliva, sputum (mucus coughed up), urine, feces, semen, vaginal secretions, and pus or other wound drainage. It does not include sweat.

Standard Precautions and Transmission-Based Precautions are a way to stop the spread of infection. They interrupt the mode of transmission. In other words, these guidelines do not stop an infected person from giving off pathogens. However, by following these two guidelines you help stop those pathogens from infecting you or those in your care:

1. Practice Standard Precautions with every single person in your care.

2. Transmission-Based Precautions vary based on how an infection is transmitted. When indicated, they are used in addition to the Standard Precautions. You will learn about these precautions in greater detail later.

Standard Precautions include the following guidelines:

Guidelines
Standard Precautions

- **Wear gloves** if you may come into contact with: blood; body fluids or secretions; broken skin (abrasions, acne, cuts, stitches, or staples); or mucous membranes (linings of the mouth, nose, eyes, vagina, rectum, and penis). Such situations include mouth care; bathroom assistance; perineal care; helping with a bedpan or urinal; cleaning up spills; cleansing basins, urinals, bedpans, and other containers that have held body fluids; and disposing of wastes.

- **Wash your hands** before putting on gloves. Wash your hands immediately after removing gloves. Be careful not to touch clean objects with your used gloves.

- **Remove gloves** immediately when finished with procedure.

- **Immediately wash all skin surfaces that have been contaminated** with blood and body fluids.

- **Wear a disposable gown** if you may come into contact with blood or body fluids.
- **Wear a mask and protective goggles** if you may come into contact with splashing or spraying blood or body fluids.
- **Wear gloves and use caution when handling razor blades, needles, and other sharps.** Sharps are needles or other sharp objects.
- **Never attempt to cap needles or sharps.** Dispose of them in an approved container.
- **Avoid nicks and cuts** when shaving residents.
- **Carefully bag all contaminated supplies.** Dispose of them according to your facility's policy.
- **Clearly label body fluids** that are being saved for a specimen with the resident's name and a biohazard label. Keep them in a container with a lid.
- **Dispose of contaminated wastes** according to your facility's policy.

Standard Precautions should ALWAYS be practiced on persons in your care regardless of their infection status. Remember, you cannot tell by how someone looks or acts, or even by reading their chart, whether they carry a bloodborne disease. If you practice Standard Precautions you greatly reduce the risk of getting a disease from those in your care. You will also keep one resident's infection from harming another.

Washing your hands is the single most important thing you can do to prevent the spread of disease! The CDC has defined **hand hygiene** as handwashing with either plain or antiseptic soap and water and using alcohol-based hand rubs. Alcohol-based hand rubs include gels, rinses, and foams. They do not require the use of water.

Alcohol-based hand rubs have proven effective in reducing bacteria on the skin. However, they are not a substitute for proper handwashing. Always use soap and water for visibly soiled hands. It is important to wash your hands often. Once they are clean, alcohol-based products can be used in addition to handwashing. Use hand lotion to prevent dry, cracked skin.

If you wear rings, consider removing them during working hours. Rings may increase the risk of contamination. Keep fingernails short and clean.

You should wash your hands:

- when you get to work
- before and after touching meal trays and/or handling food
- before and after feeding residents
- before, between, and after all contact with residents
- after contact with any body fluids
- after handling contaminated items
- before putting on gloves and after removing gloves
- before getting clean linen
- after touching garbage or trash
- after picking up anything from the floor
- before and after using the bathroom
- after blowing your nose or coughing or sneezing into your hand
- before and after you eat
- after smoking
- after touching areas on your body, such as your mouth, face, eyes, hair, ears, or nose
- before and after applying makeup
- before leaving the facility

Washing hands

Equipment: soap, paper towels

1. **Identify yourself by name. Identify the resident by name.**

2. **Turn on water at sink.**

3. **Angle arms down holding hands lower than elbows. Wet hands and wrists thoroughly (Fig. 2-28).**
   The hands are more likely to be contaminated. Water should run from cleanest to dirtiest.

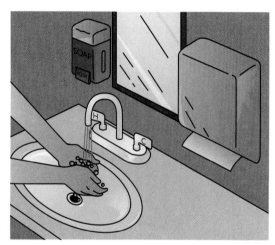

Fig. 2-28.

4. **Apply skin cleanser or soap to hands.**

5. **Lather all surfaces of hands, wrists, and fingers, producing friction, for at least 15 seconds (Fig. 2-29).**
   Lather and friction loosen skin oils and allow pathogens to be rinsed away.

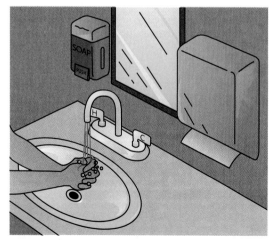

Fig. 2-29.

6. **Clean nails by rubbing them in palm of other hand.**
   Most pathogens on hands come from under nails.

7. **Rinse all surfaces of wrists, hands and fingers, keeping hands lower than the elbows and the fingertips down.**
   Wrists are cleanest, fingertips dirtiest.

8. **Use clean, dry paper towel to dry all surfaces of hands, wrists, and fingers.**

9. **Use clean, dry paper towel or knee to turn off faucet, without contaminating hands (Fig. 2-30). Do not touch the inside of the sink at any time.**
   Hands will be recontaminated if you touch the dirty faucet or sink with clean hands.

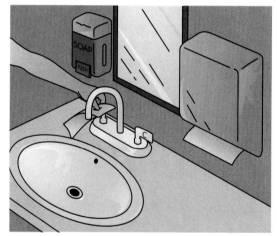

Fig. 2-30.

10. **Dispose of used paper towel(s) in wastebasket after shutting off faucet.**

👁 *When washing your hands, you must use friction for at least 15 seconds.*

Personal Protective Equipment
Personal protective equipment (**PPE**) is a barrier (a block or obstacle) between a person and disease. PPE helps protect you from potentially infectious material. PPE includes gloves, gowns, masks, goggles, and face shields. Gloves protect the hands. Gowns protect the skin and/or clothing. Masks protect the mouth and nose. Goggles protect the eyes. Face shields protect the entire face—the mouth, nose, and eyes.

Wear gloves:

- anytime you might touch blood or any body fluid, including vomitus, urine, feces, or saliva

- when performing or assisting with mouth care or care of any mucous membrane

- when performing or assisting with care of the **perineal area** (the area between and including the genitals and anus)

- when performing personal care on a resident whose skin is broken by abrasions, cuts, rash, acne, pimples, or boils

- when you have open sores or cuts on your hands

- when shaving a resident

- when disposing of soiled bed linens, gowns, dressings, and pads

Clean, non-sterile gloves are generally adequate. They may be vinyl, latex, or nitrile. Some people are allergic to latex. If you are, let the nurse know. Alternative gloves will be provided. Always let the nurse know if you have dry, cracked, or broken skin. Make sure to wash your hands before and after wearing gloves!

Disposable gloves are worn only once. They may not be washed or disinfected for reuse. Change gloves if gloves become soiled, torn, or damaged. Wash your hands before putting on fresh gloves.

Putting on gloves

1. Wash hands.

2. If right-handed, slide one glove on left hand (reverse if left-handed).

3. With gloved hand, slide other hand into the second glove.

4. Interlace fingers to smooth out folds and create a comfortable fit.

5. Carefully look for tears, holes, or spots. Replace the glove if necessary.

6. If wearing a gown, pull the cuff of the gloves over the sleeves of the gown (Fig. 2-31).

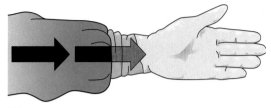

Fig. 2-31.

Remove gloves promptly after use and before caring for another resident. Wash your hands. Remove your gloves before touching non-contaminated items or surfaces.

You are wearing gloves to protect your skin from contamination. After giving care, your gloves are contaminated. If you open a door with the gloved hand, the doorknob becomes contaminated. Later, when you open the door with an ungloved hand, you will be infected. It is a common mistake to contaminate the room around you. Do not do this. Before touching surfaces, remove gloves. Wash your hands. Put on new gloves if needed.

Taking off gloves

1. Touching only the outside of one glove, pull the first glove off by pulling down from the cuff (Fig. 2-32).

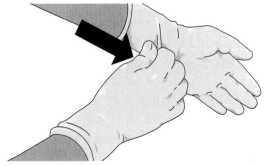

Fig. 2-32.

2. As the glove comes off the hand it should be turned inside-out.

3. With the fingertips of gloved hand hold the glove that was just removed. With ungloved hand, reach two fingers *inside* the remaining glove. Be careful not to touch any part of the outside (Fig. 2-33).

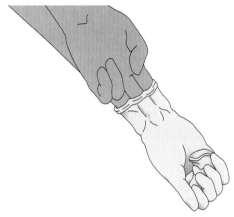

Fig. 2-33.

4. Pull down, turning this glove inside-out and over the first glove as you remove it.

5. You should now be holding one glove from its clean inner side. The other glove should be inside it.

6. Drop both gloves into the proper container.

7. Wash hands.

The guidelines for wearing other PPE are the same as for gloves. Wear PPE if there is a chance of contact with body fluids, mucous membranes, or open wounds. Gowns, masks, goggles, and face shields are worn when splashing or spraying of body fluids or blood could occur. You will decide what PPE you will need depending on the situation.

Clean, non-sterile gowns protect your exposed skin. They also prevent soiling of your clothing. When finished with a procedure, remove the gown as soon as possible. Wash your hands.

Putting on a gown

1. Wash hands.

2. Open gown. Hold out in front of you and allow gown to open. Do not shake it. Slip your arms into the sleeves. Pull gown on (Fig. 2-34).

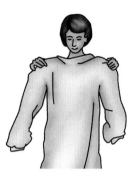

Fig. 2-34.

3. Tie the neck ties into a bow so they can be easily untied later.

4. Reaching behind, pull gown until it completely covers clothing. Tie the back ties (Fig. 2-35).

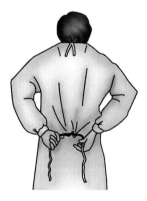

Fig. 2-35.

5. Use gowns only once and then discard or remove. When removing a gown, roll it dirty side in and away from the body. If gown becomes wet or soiled, remove it. Check clothing. Put on a new gown.

6. Put on gloves after putting on gown.

Some examiners will ask why a gown must be non-permeable. The answer is that if the clothes under the gown become wet, they are considered contaminated.

Masks should be worn when caring for residents with respiratory illnesses. Always change your mask between residents. Goggles provide protection for your eyes.

Putting on a mask and goggles

1. **Wash hands.**

2. **Pick up mask by top strings or elastic strap. Do not touch mask where it touches your face.**

3. **Adjust mask over nose and mouth. Tie top strings first, then bottom strings. Masks must always be dry or they must be replaced. Never wear a mask hanging from only the bottom tie (Fig. 2-36).**

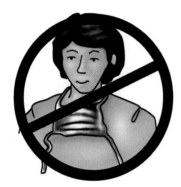

Fig. 2-36.

4. **Put on goggles.**

5. **Put on gloves *after* putting on mask and goggles.**

When additional skin protection is needed, a face shield can be used as a substitute to wearing a mask or goggles.

When applying PPE, remember this order:

1. Apply mask and goggles.

2. Apply gown.

3. Apply gloves last.

When removing PPE, remember this order:

1. Remove gloves.

2. Remove gown.

3. Remove mask and goggles.

Equipment and Linen Handling

Facilities will have separate areas for clean and dirty items, such as equipment, linen, and supplies. They are normally called the "clean" and the "dirty," or "contaminated," utility rooms. Know the location of these areas and what supplies are stored in each.

Guidelines
Handling Equipment, Linen, and Clothing

- Handle all equipment in a manner that prevents:
  - skin/mucous membrane contact
  - contamination of your clothing
  - transfer of disease to other residents or areas

- Do not use "re-usable" equipment again until it has been properly cleaned and re-processed. Measures like sterilization and disinfection decrease the spread of pathogens and disease. **Sterilization** means all microorganisms are destroyed, not just pathogens. An autoclave is usually used to sterilize equipment. It creates steam or a gas that kills all microorganisms. **Disinfection** means that only pathogens are destroyed. However, disinfection does not kill all pathogens.

- Dispose of all "single-use" equipment properly.

- Clean and disinfect:
  - all environmental surfaces
  - beds, bedrails, all bedside equipment
  - all frequently-touched surfaces (such as doorknobs)

- Handle, transport, and process soiled linens in a manner that prevents:
  - skin and mucous membrane exposure

- contamination of clothing (hold linen and clothing away from your uniform) (Fig. 2-37)

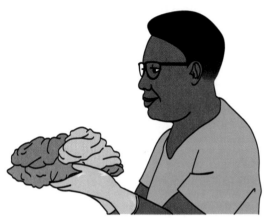

Fig. 2-37. Hold dirty linen away from your uniform.

- transfer of disease to other residents and areas (do not shake linen or clothes; fold or roll linen so that dirtiest area is inside)

You will learn more about cleaning equipment and supplies in chapter 6.

Spills

Spills can pose a serious risk of infection. Facilities will have specific cleaning solutions for spills.

Guidelines
Cleaning Spills Involving Blood, Body Fluids, or Glass

- Apply gloves before starting. In some cases, industrial-strength gloves are best.
- Clean up spills immediately with the proper cleaning solution.
- Do not pick up any pieces of broken glass, no matter how large, with your hands. Use a dustpan and broom or other tools.
- Waste containing broken glass, blood, or body fluids should be properly bagged. Put it in a trash bag and close it. Then put the first bag inside a second, clean trash bag and close it. This is called **double-bag-**

ging. Waste containing blood or body fluids may need to be placed in a special biohazard container. Follow facility policy.

Transmission-Based Precautions

These are special precautions which should be used for persons in your care who are infected or may be infected with a disease that requires additional precautions beyond Standard Precautions. They are known as Transmission-Based, or Isolation, Precautions. If approved, the new name for these precautions will be "Expanded Precautions."

There are three categories of Transmission-Based Precautions:

- Airborne Precautions
- Droplet Precautions
- Contact Precautions

The category used depends on the disease and how it spreads. They may also be used in combination for diseases that have multiple routes of transmission.

Staff often refer to residents who need these precautions as being in "isolation." A sign should be on the door indicating "isolation" or alerting people to see the nurse before entering. Two important points to remember are:

1. When indicated, Transmission-Based Precautions are always used IN ADDITION TO Standard Precautions.

2. The resident must be reassured that it is the disease, not the person with the disease, that is being isolated. Talk with your resident. Explain why these steps are being taken.

Airborne Precautions are used for diseases that can be transmitted through the air after being expelled (Fig. 2-38). The pathogens are so small that they can attach to moisture in the air. They remain floating for some time. For certain care you may be required to wear N95 or HEPA respirators to avoid infection. Airborne diseases include tuberculosis, measles, and chicken pox.

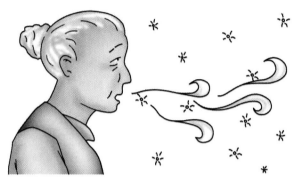

Fig. 2-38. Airborne diseases stay suspended in the air.

Droplet Precautions are used when the disease-causing microorganism does not remain in the air. They usually travel only short distances after being expelled. Droplets normally do not travel more than three feet. Droplets can be generated by coughing, sneezing, talking, laughing, or suctioning (Fig. 2-39). Droplet Precautions include wearing a face mask during care and restricting visits from uninfected people. Residents should wear masks when being moved from room to room. Cover your nose and mouth with a tissue when you sneeze or cough. Ask residents, family, and others to

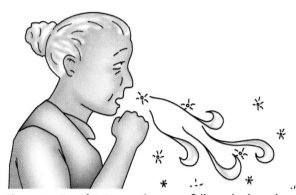

Fig. 2-39. Droplet Precautions are followed when the disease-causing microorganism does not remain in the air.

do the same. If you sneeze on your hands, wash them promptly. An example of a droplet disease is the mumps.

Contact Precautions are used when the resident is at risk of transmitting a microorganism by touching an infected object or person (Fig. 2-40). Examples include bacteria that could infect an open skin wound or infection. Lice, scabies (a skin disease that causes itching), and conjunctivitis (pink eye) are other examples. Transmission can occur during transfers or bathing. Contact Precautions include PPE and resident isolation. They require washing hands with antimicrobial soap. They also require not touching contaminated surfaces with ungloved hands or uninfected surfaces with contaminated gloves.

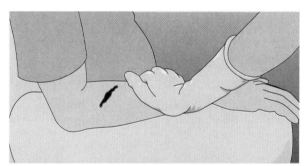

Fig. 2-40. Contact Precautions are followed when the person is at risk of transmitting a microorganism by touching an infected object or person.

Common Infectious Diseases

Bloodborne pathogens are microorganisms found in human blood. They can cause infection and disease in humans. They may also be in body fluids, draining wounds, and mucous membranes. Bloodborne diseases are transmitted by infected blood entering your bloodstream, or if infected semen or vaginal secretions contact your mucous membranes. Using a needle to inject drugs and sharing needles can also transmit bloodborne diseases. In addition, infected mothers may transmit bloodborne diseases to their babies in the womb or at birth.

In health care, contact with infectious blood or body fluids is the most common way to get a bloodborne disease. Infections can be spread through accidental contact with contaminated blood or body fluids, needles or other sharp objects, or contaminated supplies or equipment. Employers are required by law to help prevent exposure to bloodborne pathogens. The major bloodborne diseases in the United States are acquired immune deficiency syndrome (AIDS) and hepatitis. You will learn more about HIV and AIDS in chapter 8.

Hepatitis is inflammation of the liver caused by infection. Liver function can be permanently damaged by hepatitis. It can lead to other chronic, life-long illnesses. Several different viruses can cause hepatitis. The most common types of hepatitis are A, B, and C. Hepatitis B (HBV) and C are bloodborne diseases. They can cause death. HBV is a serious threat to healthcare workers. Your employer must offer you a free vaccine to protect you from hepatitis B. The HBV vaccine can prevent hepatitis B. Prevention is the best option for dealing with this disease. Take the vaccine when it is offered. There is no vaccine for hepatitis C.

Other serious infections include:

- **Tuberculosis (TB)**: TB is an airborne disease. It is carried on mucous droplets suspended in the air. TB usually infects the lungs. It causes coughing, difficulty breathing, fever, and fatigue. It can be cured. However, if left untreated, TB can cause death.

  Symptoms of TB include fatigue, loss of appetite, weight loss, slight fever and chills, night sweats, prolonged coughing, coughing up blood, chest pain, shortness of breath, and trouble breathing.

  When caring for residents who have TB, follow Standard Precautions and Airborne Precautions. Wear a mask and gown during resident care. Use special care when handling sputum. Follow isolation procedures if directed. Help the resident remember to take all medication prescribed. Failure to do so is a major factor in the spread of TB.

- **MRSA** is methicillin-resistant *Staphylococcus aureus. Staphylococcus aureus* is a common type of bacteria that can cause illness. Methicillin is a powerful antibiotic drug. MRSA is an antibiotic-resistant infection often acquired in hospitals and other facilities. MRSA can spread among those having close contact with infected people. It is almost always spread by direct physical contact, not through the air. If a person has MRSA on his skin, especially on the hands, and touches someone, he may spread MRSA. Spread also occurs through indirect contact by touching objects, such as sheets or clothes, contaminated by a person with MRSA.

  Symptoms of MRSA infection include drainage, fever, chills, and redness. Common sites include the respiratory tract, surgical wounds, perineum, rectum, and the skin. Proper handwashing, using soap and warm water, is the single most important way to control MRSA. Follow Standard Precautions.

- **VRE** is vancomycin-resistant enterococcus. Enterococcus is a bacterium that lives in the digestive and genital tracts. It does not cause problems in healthy people. Vancomycin is a powerful antibiotic. It is often the antibiotic of last resort. It is generally limited to use against bacteria that are resistant to other antibiotics. Vancomycin-resistant enterococcus is a mutant strain of enterococcus. It originally developed in people who were exposed to the antibiotic. VRE is dangerous.

It cannot be controlled with antibiotics. It causes life-threatening infections in those with weak immune systems—the very young, the very old, and the very ill. VRE is spread through direct and indirect contact.

Symptoms of VRE infection include fever, fatigue, chills, and drainage. Once it establishes itself, it is very hard to get rid of. Preventing VRE is much easier. Proper handwashing can help prevent the spread of VRE. Follow Standard Precautions.

- **Clostridium difficile (C-diff, C. difficile)** is a spore-forming bacteria which can be part of the normal intestinal flora. When the normal intestinal flora is altered, C. difficile can flourish in the intestinal tract. It produces a toxin that causes a watery diarrhea. Enemas, nasogastric tube insertion, and GI tract surgery increase a person's risk of developing the disease. The overuse of antibiotics may also alter the normal intestinal flora and increase the risk of developing C. difficile diarrhea. C. difficile can also cause colitis, a more serious intestinal condition.

C. difficile is spread by spores in feces that are difficult to kill. These spores can be carried on the hands of people who have direct contact with infected residents or with environmental surfaces (floors, bedpans, toilets, etc.) contaminated with C. difficile.

Symptoms of C. difficile include frequent, foul-smelling, watery stools. Other symptoms include diarrhea that contains blood and mucus and abdominal cramps. Proper handwashing and handling of contaminated wastes can help prevent the disease. Cleaning surfaces with an appropriate disinfectant, such as bleach, can also help. Limiting the use of antibiotics helps lower the risk of developing C. difficile diarrhea.

Employer-Employee Responsibilities

Employers' responsibilities for infection control include the following:

- Establish infection control procedures and an exposure control plan to protect workers.
- Provide continuing in-service education on infection control, including bloodborne and airborne pathogens.
- Have written procedures to follow should an exposure occur, including medical treatment and plans to prevent similar exposures.
- Provide PPE for employees to use and teach them when and how to properly use it.
- Provide free hepatitis B vaccinations for all employees.

Employees' responsibilities for infection control include the following:

- Follow Standard Precautions.
- Follow all of the facility's policies and procedures.
- Follow care plans and assignments.
- Use provided PPE as indicated or as appropriate.
- Take advantage of the free hepatitis B vaccination.
- Immediately report any exposure you have to infection.
- Participate in annual education programs covering the control of infection.

Staff have the responsibility to prevent the spread of infection. The state agency survey team will look for evidence of staff handwashing and the availability and use of personal protective equipment.

three
Understanding Your Residents

Unit 1. Explain why promoting independence and self-care is important

Any big change in lifestyle, such as moving into a nursing home, requires a huge emotional adjustment. Residents experience fear, loss, and uncertainty with their decline in health and independence. Other common reactions to illness are denial and withdrawal. All of these feelings may cause them to behave differently. Be aware that dramatic changes in a resident's life may cause anger, hostility, or depression. People handle feelings differently. Each person adjusts to illness and change in his or her own way and in his or her own time. Be supportive and encouraging. Be patient, understanding, and empathetic.

To best understand feelings residents are having, you must understand how difficult it is to lose one's independence. Somebody else must now do what residents did for themselves all of their lives. It is also difficult for friends and family members. For example, a resident may have been the main provider for his or her family. A resident may have been the person who did all of the cooking for the family.

Residents may be experiencing some of the following losses:

- loss of spouse, family members, or friends due to death
- loss of workplace and its relationships due to retirement
- loss of ability to go to favorite places
- loss of home environment and personal possessions (Fig. 3-1)

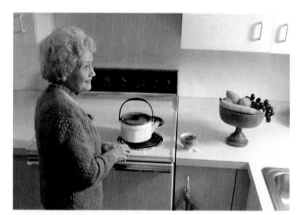

Fig. 3-1. **Understand that many residents had to leave familiar places.**

- loss of ability to attend services and meetings at their faith communities
- loss of health and the ability to care for themselves
- loss of ability to move freely
- loss of pets

Independence often means not having to rely on others for money, daily routine care, or participation in social activities. Activities of daily living (ADLs) are the personal care tasks you do every day to care for yourself. People take these activities for granted until they can no longer do them for themselves. ADLs include bathing or showering, dressing, caring for teeth and hair, toileting, eating and drinking, and moving from place to place.

A loss of independence can cause:

- a negative self-image
- anger toward caregivers, others, and self
- feelings of helplessness, sadness, and hopelessness
- feelings of being useless
- increased dependence
- depression

To prevent these feelings, encourage residents to do as much as possible for themselves. Even if it seems easier for you to do things for your residents, allow them to do tasks independently. Encourage self-care, regardless of how long it takes or how poorly they do it. Be patient (Fig. 3-2).

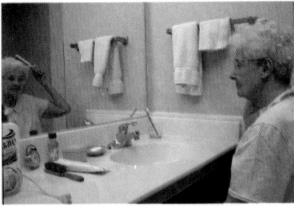

Fig. 3-2. Even if tasks take a long time, encourage residents to do what they can for themselves.

When you assist residents with their ADLs, it is important to provide respect, dignity,

and privacy. This includes the following:

- Do not interrupt them while they are in the bathroom.
- Leave the room when they receive or make personal phone calls.
- Respect their private time and personal property.
- Do not interrupt them if they are dressing themselves.
- Encourage them to do things for themselves. Be patient while they do so.
- Be patient while residents choose their clothing. Keep them covered whenever possible when you help with dressing.

RA *Never treat residents as children. They are adults. Encourage them to do self-care without rushing them. They have the right to refuse care and make their own choices. Maintaining your residents' dignity and independence is not only their legal right, but it is also the proper and ethical way for you to work.*

Unit 2. **Identify basic human needs**

People have different genes, physical appearances, cultural backgrounds, ages, and social or financial positions. But all human beings have the same basic physical needs:

- food and water
- protection and shelter
- activity
- sleep and rest
- safety
- comfort, especially freedom from pain

People also have **psychosocial needs**, which involve social interaction, emotions, intellect, and spirituality. Psychosocial needs are not as easy to define as physical needs.

However, all human beings have the following psychosocial needs:

- love and affection

- acceptance by others

- security

- self-reliance and independence in daily living

- contact with other people (Fig. 3-3)

- success and self-esteem

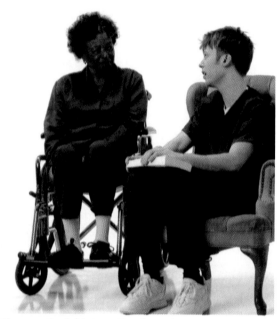

Fig. 3-3. Social interaction is an important psychosocial need.

Health and well-being affect how well psychosocial needs are met. Frustration and stress occur when basic needs are not met. This can lead to fear, anxiety, anger, aggression, withdrawal, indifference, and depression. Stress can also cause physical problems that may eventually lead to illness.

Abraham Maslow was a researcher of human behavior. He wrote about physical and psychosocial needs. He arranged these needs into an order of importance. He thought that physical needs must be met before psychosocial needs can be met. His theory is called "Maslow's Hierarchy of Needs" (Fig 3-4).

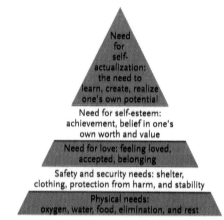

Fig. 3-4. Maslow's Hierarchy of Needs.

Humans are sexual beings. They continue to have sexual needs throughout their lives (Fig. 3-5). Sexual urges do not end due to age or admission to a nursing home. The ability to engage in sexual activity, such as intercourse and masturbation, continues unless certain diseases or injuries occur. **Masturbation** means to touch or rub sexual organs in order to give oneself or another person sexual pleasure. Sexual needs may also be affected by residents' living environments. A lack of privacy and no available partner are often reasons for a lack of sexual expression in nursing homes. Be sensitive to privacy needs.

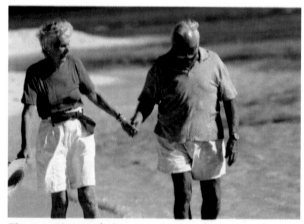

Fig. 3-5. Human beings continue to have sexual needs throughout their lives.

Residents have the right to choose how they express their sexuality. In all age groups, there is a variety of sexual behavior. This is true of your residents also. Do not judge any sexual behavior you see. An attitude that any expression of sexuality by the elderly is "disgusting" or "cute" deprives your residents of their right to dignity and respect.

Always knock or announce yourself before entering residents' rooms. Listen and wait for a response before entering. If you encounter a sexual situation between consenting adults, your role is to provide privacy and leave the room. Be open and nonjudgmental about residents' sexual attitudes. Do not judge residents' sexual orientation. Do not judge any sexual behavior you see. Honor "Do Not Disturb" signs if your facility uses them.

RR *Residents are to be protected from unwanted sexual advances of others. If you see sexual abuse happening, remove the resident from the situation. Take him or her to a safe place. Report to the nurse immediately after making sure the resident is safe and secure.*

Residents have spiritual needs. You can assist with these needs, too. Ways you can help residents with their spiritual needs include:

- If they are religious, encourage participation in religious services.
- Report to the nurse (or social worker) if a resident expresses the desire to see clergy.
- Learn about residents' religions or beliefs. Listen carefully to what your resident says.
- Respect all religious items.
- Respect residents' decisions to participate in, or refrain from, food-related rituals.
- Allow privacy for clergy and visitors (Fig. 3-6).
- If they ask you to do so, read inspirational or sacred materials aloud. If you are uncomfortable doing this, find another staff member who is not.

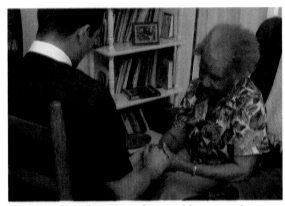

Fig. 3-6. **Be welcoming when residents receive a visit from a spiritual leader.**

You should never:

- try to change someone's religion
- tell a resident his/her belief or religion is wrong
- express judgments about a religious group
- insist a resident join religious activities
- interfere with religious practices

There are many community resources available to help residents meet different needs:

- Area Agency on Aging
- Ombudsman program
- Alzheimer's Association
- local hospice organization
- social workers
- resident advocacy organizations
- meal or transportation services

Surveyors will expect the facility to provide residents with information about community resources—especially those organizations that protect Residents' Rights.

Unit 3. **Identify ways to accommodate cultural differences**

Cultural diversity has to do with the variety of people who live and work together in the world. Positive responses to cultural diversity include acceptance and knowledge, not prejudice. Each culture may have different lifestyles, religions, customs, and behaviors.

You will take care of residents of different backgrounds and traditions other than your own. It is important to respect and value each person as an individual. Respond with acceptance. Sometimes it is easier to accept different practices or beliefs if you understand a little about them.

There are so many different cultures that they cannot all be listed here. One might talk about American culture being different from Japanese culture. But within American culture there are thousands of different groups with their own cultures. Japanese-Americans, African-Americans, and Native Americans are just a few. Even people from a particular region, state, or city can be said to have a different culture (Fig. 3-7). The culture of the South is not the same as the culture of New York City.

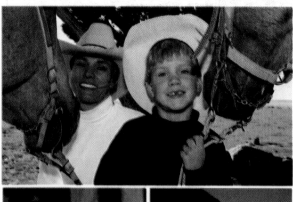
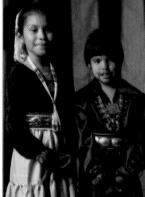
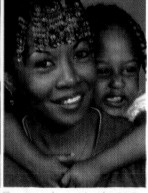

Fig. 3-7. There are many different cultures in the U.S.

Cultural background affects how friendly people are to strangers. It can affect how close they want you to stand to them when talking. Be sensitive to your residents' backgrounds. You cannot expect to be treated the same way by all your residents. You may have to adjust your behavior. Treat all residents with respect and professionalism. Expect them to treat you respectfully as well.

A resident's primary language may be different from yours. If he or she speaks a different language, an interpreter may be necessary. Take time to learn a few common phrases in a resident's native language. Picture cards and flash cards can assist with communication.

Religious differences also influence the way people behave. Religion can be very important in people's lives, particularly when they are ill or dying. You must respect the religious beliefs and practices of your residents, even if they are different from your own. Never question your residents' beliefs. Do not discuss your own beliefs with them.

Be aware of practices that affect your work with residents. Many religious beliefs include food restrictions, or rules about what and when followers can eat and drink. For example, Jewish people may not eat any pork. Be aware of any dietary restrictions and honor them. (Food differences will be discussed more in chapter 7.)

Some people's backgrounds may make them less comfortable with being touched. Be sensitive to your residents' feelings. You must touch residents in order to do your job. However, recognize that some residents feel more comfortable when there is little physical contact. If in doubt, ask residents or family members. Tell other staff members what you discover. Adjust care to your residents' needs.

Unit 4. Describe the need for activity

Activity is an essential part of a person's life. Activity improves and maintains physical and mental health. Inactivity and immobility can result in:

- loss of self-esteem
- depression
- boredom
- pneumonia
- urinary tract infection
- constipation
- blood clots
- dulling of the senses

Meaningful activities help promote independence, memory, self-esteem, and quality of life. In addition, physical activity can help manage illnesses, such as diabetes, high blood pressure, or high cholesterol. Regular physical activity can also help by:

- lessening the risk of heart disease, colon cancer, diabetes, and obesity
- relieving symptoms of depression
- improving mood and concentration
- improving body function
- lowering risk of falls
- improving sleep quality
- improving ability to cope with stress
- increasing energy
- increasing appetite and promoting better eating habits

Many facilities have an activity department. The activities are designed to help residents socialize and keep them physically and mentally active. Daily schedules are normally posted with activities for that particular day. Activities include exercise, arts and crafts, board games, newspapers, magazines, books, TV and radio, pet therapy, gardening, and group religious events.

Unit 5. Discuss family roles and their significance in health care

Families are the most important unit within our social system. Families play a huge role in most people's lives (Fig. 3-8). Some examples of family types are listed below:

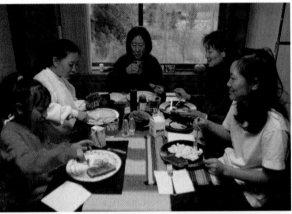
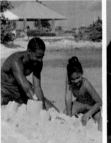
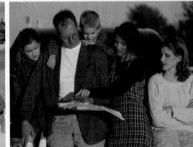

Fig. 3-8. Families come in all shapes and sizes.

- Single-parent families include one parent with a child or children.
- Nuclear families include two parents with a child or children.
- Blended families include widowed or divorced parents who have remarried. There may be children from previous marriages as well as from this marriage.
- Multigenerational families include parents, children, and grandparents.
- Extended families may include aunts, uncles, cousins, or even friends.

- Families may also be made up of unmarried couples of the same sex or opposite sexes, with or without children.

In long-term care, family members help in many ways:

- helping residents make care decisions
- communicating with the care team
- giving support and encouragement
- connecting the resident to the outside world
- offering assurance to dying residents that family memories and traditions will be valued and carried on

Be respectful and nice to friends and family members. Allow privacy for visits. After any visitor leaves, observe the effect the visit had on the resident. Report any noticeable effects to the nurse. Some residents have good relationships with their families. Others do not. If you notice any abusive behavior from a visitor towards a resident, report it immediately to the nurse.

RA *The facility has a contract with the resident to provide care 24 hours a day. Families have every right to expect quality care to continue when they cannot be with their loved one. Your obligations include the family's concerns.*

Families are great sources of information for the resident's personal preferences, history, diet, rituals, and routines. Take time to ask them questions. Families often seek out nursing assistants because they are closest to the residents. This is an important responsibility. Show families that you have time for them, too. Communicate with them, but do not discuss a resident's care with friends or family members. Listen if they want to talk. Refer questions regarding care to the nurse.

Unit 6. Describe the stages of human development

Everyone will go through the same stages of development during his or her life. However, no two people will follow the exact same pattern or rate of development. Each resident must be treated as an individual and a whole person who is growing and developing. He or she should not be treated as someone who is merely ill or disabled.

Infancy, Birth to Twelve Months

Infants grow and develop very quickly in one year. A baby moves from total dependence to the relative independence of moving around, communicating basic needs, and feeding himself.

Physical development in infancy moves from the head down. For example, infants gain control over the muscles of the neck before the muscles in their shoulders. Control over muscles in the trunk area, such as the shoulder, develops before control of arms and legs (Fig. 3-9).

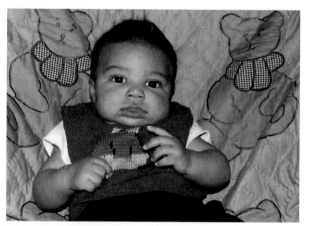

Fig. 3-9. **An infant's physical development moves from the head down.**

Childhood

The Toddler Period, Ages One to Three

During the toddler years, children gain independence. One part of this independence is new control over their bodies. Toddlers learn to speak, gain coordination of their limbs, and learn to control their bladders and bowels (Fig. 3-10).

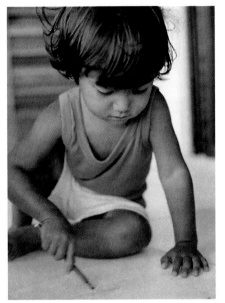

Fig. 3-10. Toddlers gain coordination of their limbs.

Toddlers assert their new independence by exploring. Poisons and other hazards, such as sharp objects, must be locked away.

Psychologically, toddlers learn that they are individuals, separate from their parents. Children of this age may try to control their parents. They may try to get what they want by throwing tantrums, whining, or refusing to cooperate. This is a key time for parents to set rules and standards.

The Preschool Years, Ages Three to Six

Children in their preschool years develop new skills. These will help them become more independent and have social relationships (Fig. 3-11). They learn new words and language skills. They learn to play in groups. They become more physically coordinated. They learn to care for themselves. Preschoolers develop ways of relating to family members. They also begin to learn right from wrong.

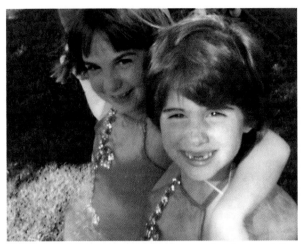

Fig. 3-11. Children in preschool years develop social relationships.

School-Age Children, Ages Six to Twelve

From ages six to about twelve years, children's development is centered on **cognitive** (related to thinking and learning) and social development. As children enter school, they also explore the world around them. They relate to other children through games, peer groups, and classroom activities. In these years, children learn to get along with each other. They also begin to behave in ways common to their sex. They begin to develop a conscience, morals, and self-esteem.

Adolescence

Puberty

During puberty, secondary sex characteristics, such as body hair, appear. Reproductive organs begin to function. The body begins to secrete reproductive hormones. The start of puberty occurs between the ages of ten and sixteen for girls and twelve and fourteen for boys.

Adolescence, Ages Twelve to Eighteen

Many teenagers have a hard time adapting to the changes that occur in their bodies after puberty. Peer acceptance is important to them. Adolescents may be afraid that they are ugly or even abnormal (Fig. 3-12).

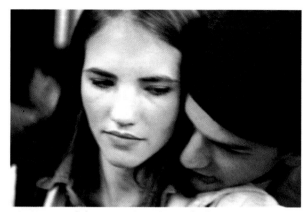

Fig. 3-12. Adolescence is a time of adapting to change.

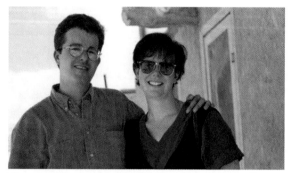

Fig. 3-13. Young adulthood often involves finding long-term mates.

This concern for body image and acceptance, combined with changing hormones that influence moods, can cause rapid mood swings. They remain dependent on their parents, but adolescents need to express themselves socially and sexually. This causes conflict and stress. Social interaction between members of the opposite sex becomes very important.

Adulthood

Each person ages in a unique way, influenced by genetics and lifestyle. Although a person cannot choose his genetic makeup, he can choose the lifestyle he leads. Habits of diet, exercise, attitude, social and physical activities, and health maintenance affect well-being later in life.

Young Adulthood, Ages Eighteen to Forty

By the age of eighteen, most young adults have stopped growing. Adopting a healthy lifestyle in these years can make life better now and prevent health problems in later adulthood. Psychological and social development continues, however. The tasks of these years include:

- selecting an appropriate education
- selecting an occupation or career
- selecting a mate (Fig. 3-13)
- learning to live with a mate or others

- raising children
- developing a satisfying sex life

Middle Adulthood: Forty to Sixty-five Years

In general, people in middle adulthood are more comfortable and stable than they were before. Many of their major life decisions have already been made. In the early years of middle adulthood people sometimes experience a "mid-life crisis." This is a period of unrest centered on a subconscious desire for change and fulfillment of unmet goals.

Late Adulthood: Sixty-five Years and Older

Persons in late adulthood must adjust to the effects of aging. These changes can include the loss of strength and health, the death of loved ones, retirement, and preparation for death. The developmental tasks of this age appear to deal entirely with loss. But solutions to these problems often involve new relationships, friendships, and interests.

Later adulthood covers an age range of as many as 25 to 35 years. People in this age category can have very different abilities, depending on their health. Some 70-year-old people enjoy active sports, while others are not active (Fig. 3-14). Many 85-year-old people can still live alone. Others may live with family members or in nursing homes.

Ideas about older people are often false. They create prejudices against the elderly.

These are as unfair as prejudices against racial, ethnic, or religious groups. On television or in the movies older people are often shown as helpless, lonely, disabled, slow, forgetful, dependent, or inactive. However, research shows that most older people are active and engaged in work, volunteer activities, and learning and exercise programs. Aging is a normal process, not a disease. Most older people live independent lives and do not need assistance (Fig. 3-15). Prejudice toward, stereotyping of, and/or discrimination against older persons or the elderly is called **ageism**.

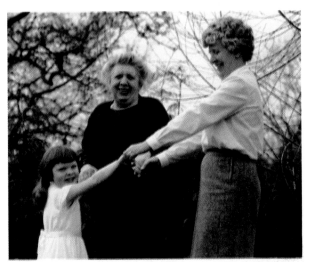

Fig. 3-14. **Most older adults often remain involved and engaged.**

As a nursing assistant you will spend much of your time working with elderly residents. You must know what is true about aging and what is not true. Aging causes many changes. *Normal changes of aging do not mean an older person must become dependent, ill, or inactive.* Knowing normal changes of aging from signs of illness or disability will allow you to better help residents.

Normal changes of aging include:

- Skin is thinner, drier, more fragile and less elastic.

- Muscles are not as strong.

- Senses of vision, hearing, taste and smell change.

- Heart works less efficiently.

- Appetite decreases.

- Elimination is more frequent.

- Hormone production changes.

- Immunity weakens.

- Mild forgetfulness occurs.

- Lifestyle changes occur.

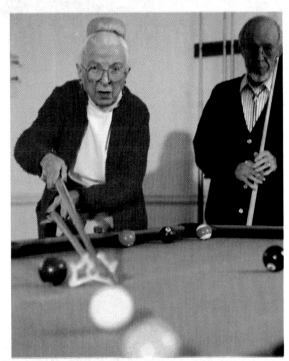

Fig. 3-15. **Most older people lead active lives.**

There are also changes that are NOT considered normal changes of aging and should be reported to the nurse. These include:

- signs of depression

- loss of ability to think logically

- poor nutrition

- shortness of breath

- incontinence

Keep in mind that this is not a complete list. *Your job includes reporting any change, normal or not.*

3

Understanding Your Residents

Unit 7. Discuss the needs of people with developmental disabilities

Some of the people you will care for will be developmentally disabled. Developmental disabilities are present at birth or emerge during childhood. A developmental disability is a chronic condition. It restricts physical or mental ability. These disabilities prevent a child from developing at a "normal" rate. Residents' care will depend on the type and the extent of the disability. A person may not be able to perform certain activities, including activities of daily living (ADLs). A person's ability to communicate may be affected. His or her ability to learn may be limited as well. Many persons with developmental disabilities require special care, treatment or other services for long periods of time or throughout their lives.

According to the CDC, mental retardation is the most common developmental disorder. Approximately 1% of the population has mental retardation. It is neither a disease nor a psychiatric illness. People with mental retardation develop at a below-average rate. They have below-average mental functioning. They experience difficulty in learning and may have problems adjusting socially.

People who are developmentally disabled require the same respect, promotion of dignity, and good care as your other residents.

Guidelines
Developmentally Disabled Residents

- Treat adult residents as adults, regardless of their behavior.

- Praise and encourage often, especially positive behavior.

- Help teach ADLs by dividing a task into smaller units.

- Promote independence. Assist residents with activities and motor functions that are difficult.

- Encourage social interaction.

- Repeat words you use to make sure they understand.

- Be patient.

Unit 8. Explain how to care for dying residents

Death can occur suddenly without warning, or it can be expected. Older people, or those with terminal illnesses, may have time to prepare for death. A **terminal illness** is a disease or condition that will eventually cause death. Preparing for death is a process. It affects the dying person's emotions and behavior.

Dr. Elisabeth Kubler-Ross studied and wrote about the process of dying. Her book, *On Death and Dying*, describes five stages of grief that dying people and their loved ones may reach before death. These five stages are listed below. Not all residents go through all the stages. They may move back and forth between stages during the process.

Denial. People in the denial stage may refuse to believe they are dying. They often believe a mistake has been made.

Anger. Once they start to face the possibility of their death, people become angry that they are dying.

Bargaining. Once people have begun to believe that they are dying, they may make promises to God. They may somehow try to bargain for their recovery.

Depression. As dying people get weaker and symptoms get worse, they may become deeply sad or depressed.

Acceptance. Many people who are dying are eventually able to accept death and prepare for it. They may make plans for their last days or for the ceremonies to follow.

Some residents will have advance directives. **Advance directives** are documents that allow people to choose what kind of medical care they wish to have if they are unable to make those decisions themselves. Advance directives can also name someone to make decisions for a person if that person becomes ill or disabled. Living Wills and Durable Power of Attorney for Health Care are examples of this. A Living Will is a written, legal document that states the medical care a person wants or does not want, in case he/she becomes unable to make those decisions him- or herself. A Durable Power of Attorney for Health Care is a legal document that appoints someone else (proxy) to make medical decisions for a person in the event he or she becomes unable to make and/or communicate such decisions personally. A "Do Not Resuscitate" (DNR) order is an order that tells medical professionals not to perform CPR. By law, advance directives and DNR orders must be honored. Be familiar with advance directives.

As with dying, grieving is an individual process. No two people will grieve in exactly the same way. Clergy, counselors, or social workers can help people who are grieving (Fig. 3-16). Family members or friends may have any of these reactions to the death of a loved one:

- shock
- denial
- anger
- guilt
- regret
- sadness
- loneliness

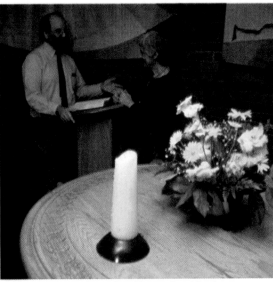

Fig. 3-16. Some people will speak with clergy to help them deal with their grief.

Death is a very sensitive topic. Many people find it hard to discuss. Feelings and attitudes about death can be formed by many factors:

- previous experiences with death
- personality type
- religious beliefs
- cultural background

RA *When a resident is dying, be considerate and respectful. Do not avoid a dying resident. Listening may be one of the most important things you can do for a resident who is dying. Provide privacy for visits from family and friends.*

Common signs of approaching death include the following:

- blurred and failing vision
- unfocused eyes
- impaired speech
- diminished sense of touch
- loss of movement, muscle tone, and feeling
- rising or below-normal body temperature
- decreasing blood pressure

- weak pulse that is abnormally slow or rapid

- slow, irregular respirations or rapid, shallow respirations, called Cheyne-Stokes respirations

- a "rattling" or "gurgling" sound as the person breathes

- cold, pale skin

- mottling, spotting, or blotching of skin caused by poor circulation

- perspiration

- incontinence (both urine and stool)

- disorientation or confusion

Guidelines
Dying Resident

- **Diminished Senses**. Reduce glare and keep room lighting low. Hearing is usually the last sense to leave the body. Speak in a normal tone. Tell them about any procedures that are being done. Observe body language to anticipate a resident's needs (Fig. 3-17).

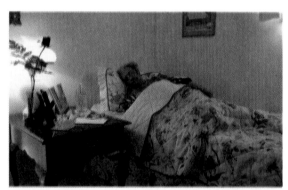

Fig. 3-17. **Keep a dying resident's room softly lit without glare.**

- **Care of the Mouth and Nose**. Give mouth care often. If the resident is unconscious, give mouth care every two hours. Apply lubricant, such as lip balm, to lips and nose.

- **Skin Care**. Give bed baths and incontinence care as needed. Bathe perspiring residents often. Skin should be kept clean and dry. Change sheets and clothes for comfort. Keep sheets wrinkle-free. Reposition residents often. Skin care to prevent pressure sores is important. (More on pressure sores is in chapter 5.)

- **Comfort**. Pain relief is critical. Observe for signs of pain, and report them. Frequent changes of position, back massage, skin care, mouth care and proper body alignment may help.

- **Environment**. Display favorite objects and photographs for resident. Make sure the room is comfortable, appropriately lit and well-ventilated.

- **Emotional and Spiritual Support**. Listening may be one of the most important things you can do for a dying resident. Touch can be very important. Some residents may seek spiritual comfort from clergy. Give privacy for visits.

You can treat residents with dignity when they are approaching death by respecting their rights and their preferences. Some legal rights to remember when caring for the terminally ill include:

1. **The right to refuse treatment.**

   Remember that whether you agree or disagree with a resident's decisions, the choice is not yours. It belongs to the person and/or his or her family. Be supportive of family members. Do not judge them. They are most likely following the resident's wishes.

2. **The right to have visitors.**

   When death is close, it is an emotional time for all those involved. Saying goodbye can be a very important part of dealing with a loved one's death.

3. **The right to privacy.**

   Privacy is a basic right, but privacy for visiting, or even when the person is alone, may be even more important now.

Other rights of a dying person are listed in Figure 3-18. Ways to treat dying residents and their families with dignity include:

I have the right to:

be treated as a living human being until I die.

maintain a sense of hopefulness, however changing its focus may be.

be cared for by those who can maintain a sense of hopefulness, however changing this might be.

express my feelings and emotions about my approaching death in my own way.

participate in decisions concerning my care.

expect continuing medical and nursing attentions even though "cure" goals must be changed to "comfort" goals.

not die alone.

be free from pain.

have my questions answered honestly.

not be deceived.

have help from and for my family in accepting my death.

die in peace and dignity.

retain my individuality and not be judged for my decisions which may be contrary to beliefs of others.

discuss and enlarge my religious and/or spiritual experiences, whatever these may mean to others.

expect that the sanctity of the human body will be respected after death.

be cared for by caring, sensitive, knowledgeable people who will attempt to understand my needs and will be able to gain some satisfaction in helping me face my death.

Fig. 3-18. The Dying Person's Bill of Rights. (This was created at a workshop on "The Terminally Ill Patient and the Helping Person," sponsored by Southwestern Michigan In-service Education Council, and appeared in the *American Journal of Nursing*, Vol. 75, January, 1975, p. 99.)

- Respect their wishes in all possible ways. Communication between staff is extremely important at this time so that everyone understands what the resident's wishes are.

- Listen carefully for ideas on how to provide simple gestures that may be special and appreciated.

- Be careful not to make promises that cannot or should not be kept.

- Listen if a dying resident wants to talk.

- Do not babble or be especially cheerful or sad. Be professional.

- Keep the resident as comfortable as possible. The nurse needs to know immediately if pain medication is requested. Keep the resident clean and dry.

- Do not isolate or avoid residents who are dying.

- Assure privacy when it is desired.

- Respect the privacy of the family and other visitors. They may be upset and not want to be bothered with others now. They may welcome a friendly smile, however, and should not be isolated, either.

- Help with the family's physical comfort. If requested, get them coffee, water, chairs, blankets, etc.

After death, the eyelids may be partially open with the eyes in a fixed stare. The jaw drops, causing the mouth to stay open. Sometimes the person may be incontinent as the muscles relax. Even though these things are a normal part of death, they can be frightening. Inform the nurse immediately to help confirm the death.

Guidelines
Postmortem Care

Postmortem care is care of the body after death. Your facility's guidelines should be followed. Only perform assigned tasks. They may include the following:

- Bathe the body. Be gentle to avoid bruising.

- Place drainage pads where needed. This is most often under the head and/or under the perineum.

- Do not remove any tubes or other equipment.

- Put dentures back in the mouth if instructed by the nurse. Close the mouth. If not possible, place dentures in denture cup near head.

- Close the eyes carefully.

- Position the body on the back with legs straight. Fold arms across the abdomen. Put a small pillow under the head.

- Follow facility policy on personal items. Check to see if you should remove jewelry. Always have a witness if personal items are removed or given to a family member. Document what was given to whom.

- Respect the wishes of family and friends. Be sensitive to their needs. If they want to sit with the body, provide privacy. Allow family members to help bathe and dress the body if they wish to do so.

- Document according to your facility's policy.

- Strip the bed after the body has been removed. Open windows to air the room, as needed. Straighten up.

Unit 9. Define the goals of a hospice program

Hospice is the term for the special care that a dying person needs. It is a compassionate way to care for dying people and their families. Hospice care uses a holistic approach. It treats the person's physical, emotional, spiritual, and social needs. Hospice care may be given in a hospital, at a care facility, or in the home. Any caregiver may give hospice care. Often specially-trained nurses, social workers and volunteers provide hospice care.

In long-term care, goals focus on recovery, or on the resident's ability to care for him- or herself as much as possible. However, in hospice care, the goals are the comfort and dignity of the resident. This type of care is called **palliative** care. This is an important difference. You will need to change your mind-set when caring for hospice residents. Focus on pain relief and comfort, rather than on teaching them to care for themselves. Report complaints or signs of pain to the nurse immediately. Residents who are dying also need to feel independent for as long as possible. Caregivers should allow residents to have as much control over their lives as possible. Eventually, caregivers may have to meet all basic needs.

Other attitudes and skills that are useful in hospice care are:

- Be a good listener, and do not feel obligated to respond. Do not push someone to talk.

- Respect privacy and independence.

- Be sensitive to individual needs. Ask family members or friends how you can be of help.

- Recognize that some persons wish to be alone with their dying loved ones.

- Be aware of your own feelings. Know your limits and respect them.

- Recognize the stress. Talking with a counselor or a support group may help.

- Take good care of yourself. Take a break when you need to.

- Allow yourself to grieve. You will develop close relationships with some residents. Know that it is normal to feel sad, angry, or lonely when residents die.

four
Body Systems

Bodies are organized into body systems. Each system has conditions under which it works best. **Homeostasis** is the condition in which all of the body's systems are balanced and are working their best. To be in homeostasis, our body's **metabolism**, or physical and chemical processes, must be working at a steady level. When disease or injury occur, the body's metabolism is disturbed. Homeostasis is lost.

Each system in the body has its own unique job. There are also normal, age-related changes for each body system. You need to understand what a normal change of aging is for each body system. This will help you better recognize any abnormal changes in your residents. This chapter also includes tips on how you can help residents with their normal changes of aging.

Body systems can be broken down in different ways. In this book we divide the human body into ten body systems:

1. Integumentary, or skin
2. Musculoskeletal
3. Nervous
4. Circulatory or Cardiovascular
5. Respiratory
6. Urinary
7. Gastrointestinal or Digestive
8. Endocrine
9. Reproductive
10. Immune and Lymphatic

Body systems are made up of organs. An organ has a specific function. Organs are made up of tissues. Tissues are made up of groups of cells that perform a similar task. For example, in the circulatory system, the heart is one of the organs. It is made up of tissues and cells. Cells are the building blocks of our bodies. Living cells divide, develop, and die, renewing the tissues and organs of our body.

This chapter discusses the structure and function, as well as age-related changes, of each body system. Diseases and disorders of each system and their care will be discussed in chapter 8.

Unit 1. Describe the integumentary system

The largest organ and system in the body is the skin (Fig. 4-1). This skin is a natural protective covering, or integument. Skin prevents injury to internal organs. It also protects the body against entry of bacteria or germs. Skin also prevents the loss of too much water, which is essential to life. Skin is made up of tissues and **glands**. Glands secrete hormones. **Hormones** are chemical substances created by the body that control numerous body functions.

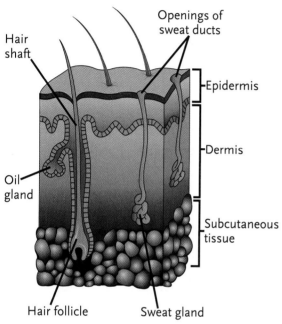

Fig. 4-1. Cross-section showing details of the integumentary system.

The skin is also a *sense* organ. It feels heat, cold, pain, touch, and pressure. It then tells the brain what it is feeling. Body temperature is controlled in the skin. Blood vessels in the skin **dilate**, or widen, when the outside temperature is too high. This brings more blood to the body surface to cool it off. The same blood vessels **constrict**, or narrow, when the outside temperature is too cold. By restricting the amount of blood reaching the skin, the blood vessels help the body retain heat.

Normal changes of aging include:

• Skin gets thinner and more fragile. It is more easily damaged.

• Skin dries and is less elastic.

• Hair thins and turns gray.

• Wrinkles and brown spots, or liver spots, appear.

• Protective fatty tissue gets thinner, so person feels colder.

• Fingernails and toenails thicken and become tougher.

How You Can Help: NA's Role

Keep residents' skin clean and dry. Use lotions as ordered for moisture. Layer clothing and bed covers for additional warmth. Keep sheets wrinkle-free. Provide careful nail care. If you are allowed to clip fingernails, do so with extreme caution. Do not cut toenails. Encourage fluids.

Observing and Reporting Integumentary System

During daily care, a resident's skin should be observed for changes that may indicate disease. Observe and report these signs and symptoms:

• rashes or flakes of dry skin

• bruising

• cuts, boils, sores, wounds

• changes in color or moistness/dryness

• swelling

• scalp or hair changes

• skin that appears different from normal or that has changed

Common Disorders Integumentary System

• Pressure sores, or decubitus ulcers (See chapter 5.)

Unit 2. Describe the musculoskeletal system

Muscles, bones, ligaments, tendons, and cartilage give the body shape and structure. They work together to move the body (Fig. 4-2). Exercise is important for improving and maintaining physical and mental health. For residents who are unable to exercise, range of motion (ROM) exercises can help. ROM exercises can prevent problems related to immobility. These problems include a loss of self-esteem, depression, pneumonia, urinary tract infections, constipation, blood clots, dulling of the senses, and muscle atrophy or contractures. When **atrophy** occurs, the muscle wastes away, decreases in size, and becomes weak. When a **contracture** develops, the muscle shortens, becomes inflexible, and "freezes" in position. This causes permanent disability of the limb. (See chapter 9 for more information on ROM exercises.)

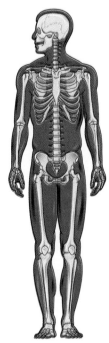

Fig. 4-2. The skeleton is composed of 206 bones that help movement and protect organs.

Normal changes of aging include:
- Muscles weaken and lose tone.
- Body movement slows.
- Joints become less flexible.
- Bones lose density. They become more brittle, making them more susceptible to breaks.
- Height is gradually lost.

4

Body Systems

How You Can Help: NA's Role

Falls can cause life-threatening complications, such as fractures. Prevent falls by keeping items out of residents' paths. Keep furniture in the same place. Keep walkers or canes where residents can easily get to them. Encourage regular movement and self-care. Assist with range of motion (ROM) exercises as needed. Position residents properly when in bed. Encourage residents to perform as many ADLs as possible.

Observing and Reporting Musculoskeletal System

Observe and report these signs and symptoms:
- changes in ability to perform routine movements and activities
- any changes in residents' ability to perform ROM exercises
- pain during movement
- any new or increased swelling of joints
- white, shiny, red, or warm areas over a joint
- bruising
- aches and pains reported to you

Common Disorders Musculoskeletal System
- Fractures
- Osteoporosis
- Arthritis
- Contractures

For more information on these disorders, see chapter 8.

Unit 3. Describe the nervous system

The nervous system is the control and message center of the body. It controls and coordinates all body functions. The nervous system also senses and interprets information from the environment outside the human body (Fig. 4-3).

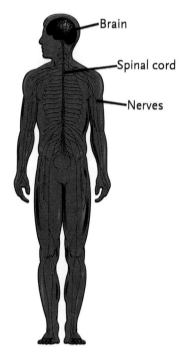

Fig. 4-3. The nervous system includes the brain, spinal cord, and nerves throughout the body.

Normal changes of aging include:

- Responses and reflexes slow.

- Sensitivity of nerve endings in skin decreases.

- Person may show some memory loss, more often with short-term memory.

How You Can Help: NA's Role

Allow plenty of time for movement. Do not rush the resident. Allow time for decision-making. Avoid sudden changes in schedule. Encourage reading and other mental activities.

Observing and Reporting
Central Nervous System

Observe and report these signs and symptoms:

- fatigue or any pain with movement or exercise

- shaking or trembling

- inability to speak clearly

- inability to move one side of body

- disturbance or changes in vision or hearing

- changes in eating patterns and/or fluid intake

- difficulty swallowing

- bowel and bladder changes

- depression or mood changes

- memory loss or confusion

- violent behavior

- any unusual or unexplained change in behavior

- decreased ability to perform ADLs

Common Disorders
Central Nervous System

- Dementias, including Alzheimer's disease and Parkinson's disease*

- Cerebrovascular accident (CVA), or stroke*

- Multiple sclerosis*

- Epilepsy

- Cerebral palsy

- Head and spinal cord injuries*

* For more information on these disorders, see chapter 8.

The Nervous System: Sense Organs

The eyes, ears, nose, tongue, and skin are the body's major sense organs (Fig. 4-4 and Fig. 4-5). They are part of the central nervous system because they receive impulses from the environment. They relay these impulses to nerves.

Normal changes of aging include:

- Vision and hearing decreases. Sense of balance may be affected.

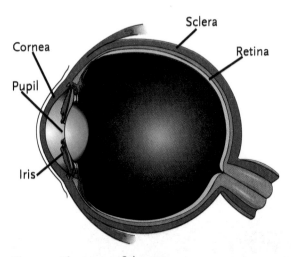

Fig. 4-4. The parts of the eye.

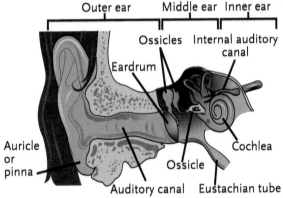

Fig. 4-5. The outer ear, middle ear, and inner ear are the three main divisions of the ear.

- Senses of taste and smell decrease.
- Sensitivity to heat and cold decreases.

How You Can Help: NA's Role

Encourage the use of eyeglasses and hearing aids. Keep them clean. Speak slowly and clearly; do not shout. Loss of senses of taste and smell may lead to decreased appetite. Encourage good oral care. Foods with a variety of tastes and textures may be provided. Loss of smell may make resident unaware of increased body odor. Assist as needed with regular bathing.

**Observing and Reporting
Eyes and Ears**

Observe and report these signs and symptoms:

- changes in vision or hearing
- signs of infection
- dizziness
- complaints of pain in eyes or ears

**Common Disorders
Eyes and Ears**

- Cataracts
- Glaucoma
- Deafness

Unit 4. **Describe the circulatory or cardiovascular system**

The circulatory system is made up of the heart, blood vessels, and blood. The heart pumps blood through the blood vessels to the cells. The blood carries food, oxygen, and other substances cells need to function properly (Fig. 4-6).

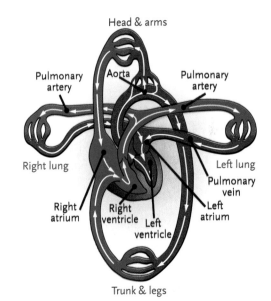

Fig. 4-6. The flow of blood through the heart.

The circulatory system performs these major functions:

- supplying food, oxygen, and hormones to cells
- producing and supplying infection-fighting blood cells
- removing waste products from cells
- controlling body temperature

4

Body Systems

Normal changes of aging include:

- Heart muscle loses strength.
- Blood vessels narrow.
- Blood flow decreases.

How You Can Help: NA's Role

Encourage movement and exercise. Allow enough time to complete activities. Prevent residents from tiring. Keep legs and feet warm.

Observing and Reporting
Circulatory System

Observe and report these signs and symptoms:

- changes in pulse rate
- weakness, fatigue
- loss of ability to perform activities of daily living (ADLs)
- swelling of hands and feet
- pale or bluish hands, feet, or lips
- chest pain
- weight gain
- shortness of breath, changes in breathing patterns, inability to catch breath
- severe headache
- inactivity (which can lead to circulatory problems)

Common Disorders
Circulatory System

- Hardening and narrowing of the blood vessels
- Myocardial infarction (MI), or heart attack*
- Angina pectoris*
- Hypertension, or high blood pressure*
- Congestive heart failure*
- Peripheral vascular disease*

* For more information on these disorders, see chapter 8.

Unit 5. **Describe the respiratory system**

Respiration, the body taking in oxygen and removing carbon dioxide, involves breathing in (**inspiration**), and breathing out (**expiration**). The lungs accomplish this process (Fig. 4-7).

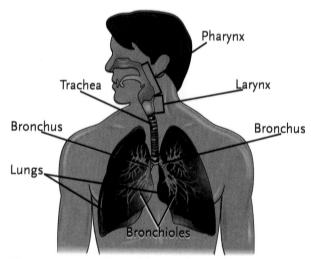

Fig. 4-7. An overview of the respiratory system.

The respiratory system has two functions:

1. It brings oxygen into the body.
2. It eliminates carbon dioxide produced as the body uses oxygen.

Normal changes of aging include:

- Lung strength decreases.
- Lung capacity decreases.
- Oxygen in the blood decreases.
- Voice weakens.

How You Can Help: NA's Role

Encourage residents to get out of bed often. Encourage exercise and regular movement. Encourage and assist with deep breathing exercises.

Observing and Reporting
Respiratory System

Observe and report these signs and symptoms:

- change in respiratory rate
- shallow breathing or breathing through pursed lips
- coughing or wheezing
- nasal congestion or discharge
- sore throat, difficulty swallowing, or swollen tonsils
- the need to sit after mild exertion
- pale or bluish color of the lips and arms and legs
- pain in the chest area
- discolored **sputum**, or the fluid a person coughs up (green, yellow, blood-tinged, or gray)

Common Disorders
Respiratory System

- Asthma
- Upper respiratory infection (URI), or a cold
- Bronchitis*
- Pneumonia*
- Emphysema*
- Lung cancer
- Tuberculosis
- Chronic Obstructive Pulmonary Disease (COPD)*

* For more information on these disorders, see chapter 8.

Unit 6. Describe the urinary system

The urinary system has two functions:

1. It eliminates waste products created by the cells through urine.

2. It maintains water balance in the body.

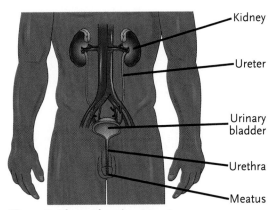

Fig. 4-8. The male urinary system.

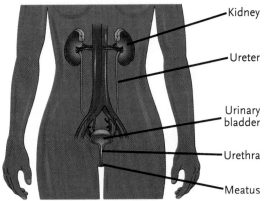

Fig. 4-9. The female urinary system. The female urethra is shorter than the male urethra. Because of this, the female bladder is more likely to become infected by bacteria traveling up the urethra. Encourage female residents to wipe from front to back after elimination. When you give perineal care, make sure you do this as well.

Normal changes of aging include:

- The ability of kidneys to filter blood decreases.
- Bladder muscle tone weakens.
- Bladder holds less urine, which causes more frequent urination.
- Bladder may not empty completely, causing more susceptibility to infection.

How You Can Help: NA's Role

Encourage residents to drink fluids. Offer frequent trips to the bathroom. If residents are incontinent, do not show frustration or anger. Keep residents clean and dry.

4

Body Systems

Observing and Reporting
Urinary System

Observe and report these symptoms:

- weight loss or gain

- swelling in upper or lower extremities

- pain or burning during urination

- changes in urine, such as cloudiness, odor, or color

- changes in frequency and amount of urination

- swelling in the abdominal/bladder area

- complaints that bladder feels full or painful

- incontinence/dribbling

- pain in the kidney or back/flank region

- inadequate fluid intake

Common Disorders
Urinary System

- Urinary tract infection (UTI), or cystitis*

- Calculi (kidney stones)

- Nephritis

- Renovascular hypertension

- Chronic kidney failure

* For more information on this disorder, see chapter 8.

Unit 7. Describe the gastrointestinal or digestive system

The gastrointestinal (GI) system, also called the digestive system (Fig. 4-10), has two functions:

1. **Digestion** is the process of breaking down food so that it can be absorbed into the cells.

2. **Elimination** is the process of expelling solid wastes that are not absorbed into the cells.

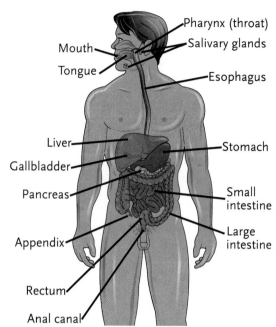

Fig. 4-10. The GI system consists of all the organs needed to digest food and process waste.

Normal changes of aging include:

- Saliva and digestive fluids decrease.

- Difficulty chewing and swallowing may occur.

- Absorption of vitamins and minerals decreases.

- Process of digestion is less efficient, causing more frequent constipation.

How You Can Help: NA's Role

Encourage fluids and nutritious, appealing meals. Allow time to eat. Make mealtime enjoyable. Provide good oral care. Make sure dentures fit properly and are cleaned regularly. Encourage daily bowel movements. Give residents the opportunity to have a bowel movement around the same time each day.

Observing and Reporting
Gastrointestinal System

Observe and report these symptoms:

- difficulty swallowing or chewing (including denture problems, tooth pain, or mouth sores)

- fecal incontinence (losing control of bowels)

- weight gain/weight loss
- anorexia (loss of appetite)
- abdominal pain and cramping
- diarrhea
- nausea and vomiting (especially vomitus that looks like coffee grounds)
- constipation
- gas
- hiccups, belching
- bloody, black, or hard stool
- heartburn
- poor nutritional intake

Common Disorders
Gastrointestinal System

- Peptic ulcers
- Hepatitis
- Ulcerative colitis
- Colorectal cancer
- Hemorrhoids*

* For more information on this disorder, see chapter 8.

Unit 8. Describe the endocrine system

The endocrine system is made up of glands that secrete hormones. Hormones are chemicals that control many of the organs and body systems (Fig. 4-11). Hormones are carried in blood to the organs. Hormones regulate the body processes, including:

- maintaining homeostasis
- influencing growth and development
- regulating levels of sugar in the blood
- regulating levels of calcium in the bones
- regulating the body's ability to reproduce
- determining how fast cells burn food for energy

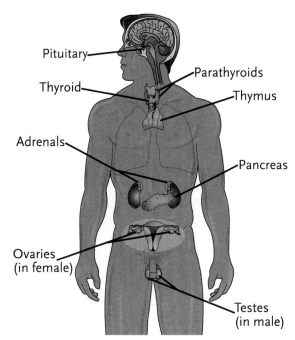

Fig. 4-11. The endocrine system includes organs that produce hormones that regulate body processes.

Normal changes of aging include:

- Levels of hormones, such as estrogen and progesterone, decrease.
- Insulin production lessens.
- Body is less able to handle stress.

How You Can Help: NA's Role

*Encourage proper nutrition. Remove or reduce stressors. **Stressors** are anything that causes stress. Offer encouragement and listen to residents.*

Observing and Reporting
Endocrine System

Many endocrine illnesses can be treated with hormone supplements. These supplements must be given very precisely. For example, too much insulin administered to a diabetic can cause the sudden start of insulin shock.

Observe and report these symptoms:

- headache*
- weakness*
- blurred vision*

- dizziness*
- hunger*
- irritability*
- sweating/excessive perspiration*
- change in "normal" behavior*
- increased confusion*
- weight gain/weight loss
- loss of appetite/increased appetite
- increased thirst
- frequent urination
- dry skin
- sluggishness or fatigue
- hyperactivity

* indicates signs and symptoms that should be reported immediately

Common Disorders
Endocrine System

- Hyperthyroidism
- Hypothyroidism
- Diabetes mellitus*

* For more information, see chapter 8.

Unit 9. Describe the reproductive system

The reproductive system is made up of the reproductive organs. They are different in men and women (Fig. 4-12 and Fig. 4-13). The reproductive system allows human beings to **reproduce**, or create new human life. Reproduction begins when a male's and female's sex cells (sperm and ovum) join. These sex cells are formed in the male and female sex glands. These sex glands are called the gonads.

Normal changes of aging include:

Female:

- Menstruation ends.

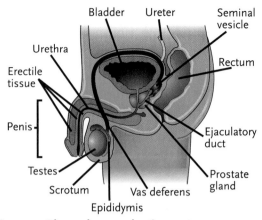

Fig. 4-12. The male reproductive system.

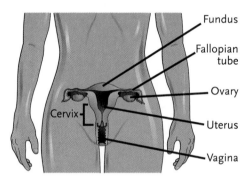

Fig. 4-13. The female reproductive system.

- Decrease in estrogen leads to loss of calcium. This causes brittle bones and, potentially, osteoporosis.
- Vaginal walls become drier and thinner.

Male:

- Sperm production decreases.
- Prostate gland enlarges, which can interfere with urination.

How You Can Help: NA's Role

Sexual needs continue as people age. Provide privacy whenever necessary for sexual activity. Respect your residents' sexual needs. Never make fun of or judge any sexual behavior.

RA *Residents have the right to sexual freedom and expression. Residents have the right to privacy and to meet their sexual needs.*

Observing and Reporting
Reproductive System

Observe and report these symptoms:

- discomfort or difficulty with urination
- discharge from the penis or vagina
- swelling of the genitals
- blood in urine or stool
- breast changes, including size, shape, lumps, or discharge from the nipple
- sores on the genitals
- resident reports impotence, or inability of male to have sexual intercourse
- resident reports painful intercourse

Common Disorders
Reproductive System

- Breast, prostate*, and ovarian cancer
- Vaginitis*

* For more information on these disorders, see chapter 8.

Unit 10. Describe the immune and lymphatic systems

The immune system protects the body from disease-causing bacteria, viruses, and organisms. The immune system protects the body in two ways:

1. Nonspecific immunity protects the body from disease in general.

2. Specific immunity protects against a particular disease that is invading the body at a given time.

The lymphatic system removes excess fluids and waste products from the body's tissues. It also helps the immune system fight infection (Fig. 4-14). It is closely related to both the immune and the circulatory systems. The lymphatic system consists of lymph vessels and lymph capillaries in which a fluid called lymph circulates. Lymph is a clear yellowish fluid that carries disease-fighting cells called lymphocytes.

Normal changes of aging include:
- Increased risk of all types of infections
- Decreased response to vaccines

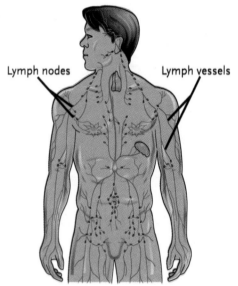

Fig. 4-14. Lymph nodes work to fight infection and are located throughout the body.

How You Can Help: NA's Role

Factors that weaken the immune system include not enough sleep, poor nutrition, chronic illness, and stress. Follow rules for preventing infection. Wash hands often. Keep the resident's environment clean to prevent infection. Encourage and help with good personal hygiene. Encourage proper nutrition and fluid intake. Promote a comfortable environment that allows for enough rest.

Observing and Reporting
Immune and Lymphatic Systems

Observe and report these symptoms:

- recurring infections (such as fevers and diarrhea)
- swelling of the lymph nodes
- increased fatigue

Common Disorders
Immune System

- HIV/AIDS*
- Lymphoma

* For more information, see chapter 8.

five

Personal Care Skills

Unit 1. Explain personal care of residents

Hygiene is the term used to describe ways to keep bodies clean and healthy. Bathing and brushing teeth are two examples. Grooming means practices like caring for fingernails and hair. Hygiene and grooming, as well as dressing and eating, are called activities of daily living (ADLs). You will help residents every day with these tasks. These activities are often referred to as "A.M. care" or "P.M. care." This refers to the time of day they are performed.

A.M. care includes the following:

- offering a bedpan or urinal or assisting the resident to the bathroom

- assisting the resident to wash face and hands

- helping with mouth care before or after breakfast, as the resident prefers

P.M. care includes the following:

- offering a bedpan or urinal or helping the resident to the bathroom

- helping the resident to wash face and hands

- giving a snack (if allowed)

- performing mouth care

- giving a back rub (if allowed)

The way you help residents with personal care plays a large part in promoting their independence and dignity. The tasks you help with and how much help you give will be different for each resident. It will depend on each resident's ability to do self-care and/or his or her physical or mental limitations. For example, a resident who has recently had a stroke will need more help than one who has a broken foot that is almost healed. Promoting independence is an important part of the care you give.

Personal care is a very private experience. It may be embarrassing for some residents. You must be professional when helping with these tasks. Before you begin, explain to the resident exactly what you will be doing. Ask if he or she would like to use the bathroom or bedpan first. Provide the resident with privacy. Let him or her make as many decisions as possible about when, where, and how a procedure is done (Fig. 5-1). This promotes dignity and independence. Encourage a resident to do as much as he or she is able to do while giving care.

During personal care, look for any problems or changes that have occurred. Personal care gives you a chance to talk with residents. Some residents will share feelings and concerns with you. Look for physical and mental changes. You can also observe a resident's environment. Look for unsafe or unhealthy surroundings. Report these to the nurse.

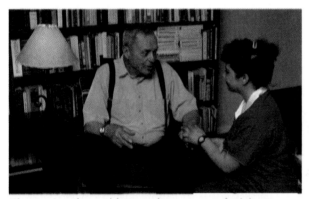

Fig 5-1. Let the resident make as many decisions as possible about the personal care you will perform.

If the resident seems tired, stop and take a short rest. Never rush him or her. After care, always ask if the resident would like anything else. Leave the resident's area clean and tidy. Make sure the call light is within reach. Leave the bed in its lowest position unless instructed otherwise.

Observing and Reporting
Personal Care

- skin-color, temperature, redness (more information listed in unit 7)
- mobility
- flexibility
- comfort level, or complaints of pain or discomfort
- strength and the ability to perform self-care and ADLs
- mental and emotional state
- resident complaints

Unit 2. Describe guidelines for assisting with bathing

Bathing promotes good health and well-being. It removes perspiration, dirt, oil, and dead skin cells from the skin. Bathing gives you a chance to observe a resident's skin. For bed-bound residents, bed baths will move arms and legs. This increases body movement and circulation.

Guidelines
Bathing

- The face, hands, underarms, and perineum should be washed every day. The **perineum** includes the genitals and anus and the area between them. A complete bath or shower can be taken every other day or even less often.

- Older skin produces less perspiration and oil. Elderly people with dry and fragile skin should bathe only once or twice a week. This prevents further dryness.

- Use only products approved by the facility or that the resident prefers.

- Before any bathing task, make sure the room is warm enough.

- Before bathing, make sure the water temperature is safe and comfortable. Test the water temperature to make sure it is not too hot. Then have the resident test the water temperature. The resident is best able to choose a comfortable water temperature.

- Gather supplies before giving a bath so the resident is not left alone.

- Make sure all soap is removed from the skin before completing the bath.

- Keep a record of the bathing schedule for each resident. Follow the care plan.

Giving a complete bed bath

Equipment: bath blanket, bath basin, soap, bath thermometer, 2-4 washcloths, 2-4 bath towels, clean gown or clothes, gloves, lotion, deodorant, orangewood stick or emery board

1. **Wash hands.**
   Provides for infection control.

2. **Identify yourself by name. Identify the resident by name.**
   Resident has right to know identity of his or her caregiver. Addressing resident by name shows respect and establishes correct identification.

3. **Explain procedure to resident. Speak clearly, slowly, and directly. Maintain face-to-face contact whenever possible.**
   Promotes understanding and independence.

4. **Provide for resident's privacy with curtain, screen, or door. Be sure the room is at a comfortable temperature and there are no drafts.**
   Maintains resident's right to privacy and dignity.

5. **Adjust bed to a safe working level, usually waist high. Lock bed wheels.**
   Prevents injury to you and to resident.

6. **Adjust position of side rails to ensure resident safety at all times.**

7. **Place a bath blanket or towel over resident (Fig. 5-2). Ask him to hold onto it as you remove or fold back top bedding. Keep resident covered with bath blanket (or top sheet).**

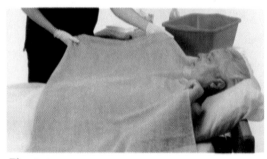

Fig. 5-2.

8. **Fill the basin with warm water. Test water temperature with thermometer or your wrist and ensure it is safe. Water temperature should be 105° to 110° F. It cools quickly. Have resident check water temperature. Adjust if necessary. Change the water when it becomes too cool, soapy, or dirty.**
   Resident's sense of touch may be different than yours; therefore, resident is best able to identify a comfortable water temperature.

9. **If resident has open wounds, put on gloves.**
   Protects you from contact with body fluids.

10. **Ask and help resident to participate in washing.**
    Promotes independence.

11. **Uncover only one part of the body at a time. Place a towel under the body part being washed.**
    Promotes resident's dignity and right to privacy. Also helps keep resident warm.

12. **Wash, rinse, and dry one part of the body at a time. Start at the head. Work down, and complete the front first. Fold the washcloth over your hand like a mitt and hold it in place with your thumb (Fig. 5-3).**

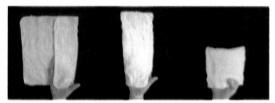

Fig. 5-3.

Eyes and Face: **Wash face with wet washcloth (no soap). Begin with the eye farther away from you. Wash inner aspect to outer aspect (Fig. 5-4). Use a different area of the washcloth for each eye. Wash the face from the middle outward. Use firm but gentle strokes. Wash the neck and ears and behind the ears. Rinse and pat dry.**

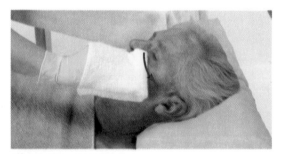

Fig. 5-4.

Arms: **Remove the resident's top clothing. Cover him with the bath blanket or** towel. With a soapy washcloth, wash the upper arm and underarm. Use long strokes from the shoulder to the elbow. Rinse and pat dry. Wash the elbow. Wash, rinse, and dry from the elbow down to the wrist (Fig. 5-5).

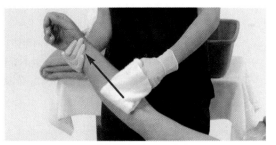

Fig. 5-5.

Wash the hand in a basin. Clean under the nails with an orangewood stick or nail brush (Fig. 5-6). Rinse and pat dry. Give nail care (see procedure later in this chapter) if it has been assigned. Repeat for the other arm. Put lotion on the resident's elbows and hands if ordered.

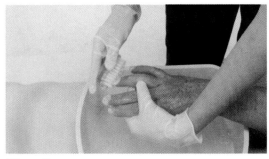

Fig. 5-6.

Chest: Place the towel across the resident's chest. Pull the blanket down to the waist. Lift the towel only enough to wash the chest. Rinse it and pat dry. For a female resident, wash, rinse, and dry breasts and under breasts. Check the skin in this area for signs of irritation.

Abdomen: Fold the blanket down so that it still covers the pubic area. Wash the abdomen, rinse, and pat dry. Cover with the towel. Pull the cotton blanket up to the resident's chin. Remove the towel.

Legs and Feet: Expose one leg. Place a towel under it. Wash the thigh. Use long downward strokes. Rinse and pat dry. Do the same from the knee to the ankle (Fig. 5-7).

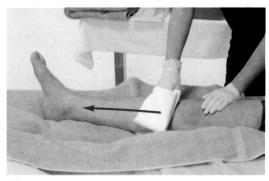

Fig. 5-7.

Place another towel under the foot. Move the basin to the towel. Place the foot into the basin. Wash the foot and between the toes (Fig. 5-8). Rinse foot and pat dry. Give nail care (see procedure later in this chapter) if it has been assigned. Do not give nail care for a diabetic resident. Never clip a resident's toenails. Apply lotion to the foot if ordered, especially at the heels. Do not apply lotion between the toes. Repeat steps for the other leg and foot.

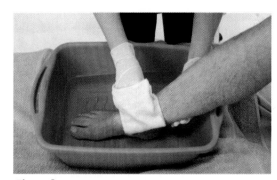

Fig. 5-8.

Back: Help resident move to the center of the bed. Ask resident to turn onto his side so his back is facing you. If the bed has rails, raise the rail on the far side for safety. Fold the blanket away from the back. Place a towel lengthwise next to the back. Wash the back, neck, and but-

5

Personal Care Skills

5

Personal Care Skills

tocks with long, downward strokes. Rinse and pat dry (Fig. 5-9). Apply lotion if ordered.

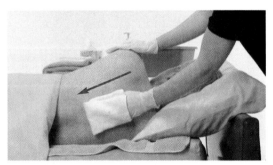

Fig. 5-9.

13. Place the towel under the buttocks and upper thighs. Help the resident turn onto his back. If the resident is able to wash his or her perineal area, place a basin of clean, warm water and a washcloth and towel within reach. Leave the room if the resident desires. If the resident has a urinary catheter in place, remind him not to pull it.

14. If the resident cannot provide perineal care, you must do so. Put on gloves (if you haven't already done so) first. Provide privacy at all times.

15. Change bath water. Wash, rinse, and dry perineal area. Work from front to back.

    For a female resident: Wash the perineum with soap and water from *front to back*. Use single strokes (Fig. 5-10).

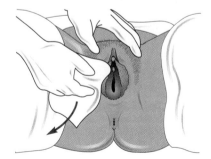

Fig. 5-10.

Do not wash from the back to the front, as this may cause infection. Use a clean area of washcloth or clean washcloth for each stroke. First wipe the center of the perineum, then each side. Then spread the labia majora, the outside folds of perineal skin that protect the urinary meatus and the vaginal opening. Wipe from front to back on each side. Rinse the area in the same way. Dry entire perineal area. Move from front to back. Use a blotting motion with towel. Ask resident to turn on her side. Wash, rinse, and dry buttocks and anal area. Clean the anal area without contaminating the perineal area.

For a male resident: If the resident is uncircumcised, pull back the foreskin first. Gently push skin towards the base of penis. Hold the penis by the shaft. Wash in a circular motion from the tip down to the base. Use a clean area of washcloth or clean washcloth for each stroke (Fig. 5-11).

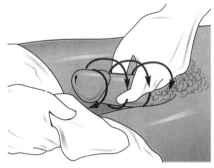

Fig. 5-11.

Rinse the penis. If resident is uncircumcised, gently return foreskin to normal position. Then wash the scrotum and groin. The groin is the area from the pubis (area around the penis and scrotum) to the upper thighs. Rinse and pat dry. Ask the resident to turn on his side. Wash, rinse, and dry buttocks and anal area. Clean the anal area without contaminating the perineal area.

16. Provide deodorant.

17. Remove and dispose of gloves properly.

18. **Put clean gown on resident. Assist with brushing or combing resident's hair (see procedure later in the chapter).**

19. **Make resident comfortable. Replace bedding.**

20. **Return bed to appropriate position. Remove privacy measures.**
    Lowering the bed provides for safety.

21. **Put call light within resident's reach.**
    Call light allows resident to communicate with staff as necessary.

22. **Place soiled clothing and linens in proper containers.**

23. **Empty, rinse, and wipe bath basin. Return to proper storage.**

24. **Wash hands.**
    Provides for infection control.

25. **Report any changes in resident to the nurse.**
    Provides nurse with information to assess resident.

26. **Document procedure using facility guidelines.**
    What you write is a legal record of what you did. If you don't document it, legally it didn't happen.

A partial bath is done on days when a complete bed bath, tub bath, or shower is not done. It includes washing the face, underarms, and hands, and performing perineal care.

Shampooing in bed

Equipment: shampoo, hair conditioner if requested, 2 bath towels, washcloth, bath thermometer, pitcher or hand-held shower or sink attachment, waterproof pad, bath blanket, trough, basin, comb and brush, hair dryer

1. **Wash hands.**
   Provides for infection control.

2. **Identify yourself by name. Identify the resident by name.**
   Resident has right to know identity of his or her caregiver. Addressing resident by name shows respect and establishes correct identification.

3. **Explain procedure to resident. Speak clearly, slowly, and directly. Maintain face-to-face contact whenever possible.**
   Promotes understanding and independence.

4. **Provide for resident's privacy with curtain, screen, or door. Make sure room is at a comfortable temperature and there are no drafts.**
   Maintains resident's right to privacy and dignity.

5. **Adjust bed to a safe working level, usually waist high. Lock bed wheels.**
   Prevents injury to you and to resident.

6. **Lower head of bed. Remove pillow.**

7. **Test water temperature with thermometer or your wrist. Ensure it is safe. Water temperature should be 105° F. Have resident check water temperature. Adjust if necessary.**
   Resident's sense of touch may be different than yours; therefore, resident is best able to identify a comfortable water temperature.

8. **Raise the side rail farthest from you.**

9. **Place the waterproof pad under the resident's head and shoulders. Cover the resident with the bath blanket. Fold back the top sheet and regular blankets.**
   Protects bed linen.

10. **Place collection container (e.g., trough, basin) under resident's head. Place one towel across the resident's shoulders.**

11. **Protect resident's eyes with dry washcloth.**

12. **Use pitcher or attachment to wet hair thoroughly. Apply a small amount of shampoo.**

13. **Lather and massage scalp with fingertips (Fig. 5-12). Use a circular motion from front to back. Do not scratch the scalp.**

5

Personal Care Skills

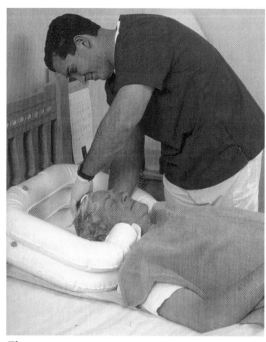

Fig. 5-12.

14. **Rinse hair until water runs clear. Apply conditioner. Rinse as directed on container.**

15. **Cover resident's hair with clean towel. Dry his face with washcloth used to protect eyes.**

16. **Remove trough and waterproof covering.**

17. **Raise head of bed.**

18. **Gently rub the scalp and hair with the towel.**

19. **Dry and comb resident's hair as he or she prefers. See procedure later in the chapter.**

20. **Return bed to appropriate level. Remove privacy measures.**

    Lowering the bed provides for safety.

21. **Before leaving, place call light within resident's reach.**

    Allows resident to communicate with staff as necessary.

22. **Empty, rinse, and wipe bath basin/pitcher. Return to proper storage.**

23. **Clean comb/brush. Return hair dryer and comb/brush to proper storage.**

24. **Place soiled linen in proper container.**

25. **Wash hands.**

    Provides for infection control.

26. **Report any changes in resident to nurse.**

    Provides nurse with information to assess resident.

27. **Document procedure using facility guidelines.**

    What you write is a legal record of what you did. If you don't document it, legally it didn't happen.

Many people prefer showers or tub baths to bed baths (Fig. 5-13 and Fig. 5-14). Check with the nurse first to make sure a shower or tub bath is allowed.

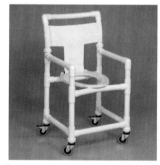

Fig. 5-13. A shower chair assists residents who take showers.

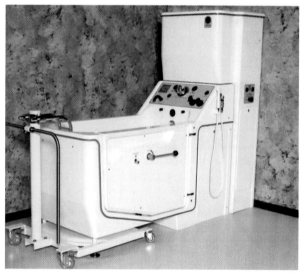

Fig. 5-14. A common style of tub in nursing homes. (Photo courtesy of Lee Penner of Penner Tubs)

Guidelines
Safety for Showers and Tub Baths

• Clean tub or shower before and after use.

- Make sure bathroom or shower room floor is dry.

- Be familiar with available safety and assistive devices. Check that hand rails, grab bars, and lifts are in working order.

- Have resident use safety bars when getting into or out of the tub or shower.

- Some facilities have a policy that requires you to undress residents in their rooms before moving them to the shower room. If so, cover resident while transporting to and from shower or tub room. It provides warmth and privacy. In other facilities, policy requires you to move residents to the shower room and undress them there.

- Place all needed items within reach.

- Do not leave resident alone.

- Avoid using bath oils. They make surfaces slippery.

- Test water temperature with thermometer or your wrist before resident gets into shower. Water temperature should be no more than 105° F. Make sure temperature is comfortable for resident.

RA *Privacy is very important when transporting residents to the shower or tub room and during the shower or tub bath. Make sure the body is not unnecessarily exposed.*

Giving a shower or a tub bath

Equipment: bath blanket, soap, shampoo, bath thermometer, 2-4 washcloths, 2-4 bath towels, clean gown and robe or clothes, non-skid footwear, gloves, lotion, deodorant

1. **Wash hands.**
   Provides for infection control.

2. **Place equipment in shower or tub room. Clean shower or tub area and shower chair.**
   Reduces pathogens and prevents the spread of infection.

3. **Wash hands.**
   Provides for infection control.

4. **Go to resident's room. Identify self by name. Identify resident by name.**
   Resident has right to know identity of his or her caregiver. Addressing resident by name shows respect and establishes correct identification.

5. **Explain procedure to resident. Speak clearly, slowly, and directly. Maintain face-to-face contact whenever possible.**
   Promotes understanding and independence.

6. **Provide for resident's privacy with curtain, screen, or door.**
   Maintains resident's right to privacy and dignity.

7. **Help resident to put on nonskid footwear. Transport resident to shower or tub room.**
   Nonskid footwear helps lessen the risk of falls.

For a shower:

8. **If using a shower chair, place it into position. Lock wheels. Safely transfer resident into shower chair.**
   Chair may slide if resident attempts to get up.

9. **Turn on water. Test water temperature with thermometer. Water temperature should be no more than 105° F. Have resident check water temperature.**
   Resident's sense of touch may be different than yours; therefore, resident is best able to identify a comfortable water temperature.

For a tub bath:

8. **Safely transfer resident onto chair or tub lift.**

9. **Fill the tub halfway with warm water. Test water temperature with thermometer. Water temperature should be no more than 105° F. Have resident check water temperature.**

Remaining steps for either procedure:

10. **Put on gloves.**
    Protects you from contact with body fluids.

11. **Help resident remove clothing and shoes.**

5

Personal Care Skills

12. **Help the resident into shower or tub. Put shower chair into shower and lock wheels.**

13. **Stay with resident during procedure.**
    Provides for resident's safety.

14. **Let resident wash as much as possible. Assist to wash his or her face.**
    Encourages resident to be independent.

15. **Help resident shampoo and rinse hair.**

16. **Help to wash and rinse the entire body. Move from head to toe.**

17. **Turn off water or drain the tub. Cover resident with bath blanket until the tub drains.**
    Maintains resident's dignity and right to privacy by not exposing body. Keeps resident warm.

18. **Unlock shower chair wheels if used. Roll resident out of shower, or help resident out of tub and onto a chair.**

19. **Give resident towel(s) and help to pat dry. Remember to pat dry under the breasts, between skin folds, in the perineal area, and between toes.**
    Patting dry prevents skin tears and reduces chafing.

20. **Apply lotion and deodorant as needed.**

21. **Place soiled clothing and linens in proper containers.**

22. **Remove gloves and dispose of them.**

23. **Wash hands.**
    Provides for infection control.

24. **Help resident dress and comb hair before leaving shower or tub room. Put on non-skid footwear. Return resident to room.**
    Combing hair in shower room allows resident to maintain dignity when returning to room.

25. **Make sure resident is comfortable.**

26. **Before leaving, place call light within resident's reach.**
    Allows resident to communicate with staff as necessary.

27. **Report any changes in resident to nurse.**
    Provides nurse with information to assess resident.

28. **Document procedure using facility guidelines.**
    What you write is a legal record of what you did. If you don't document it, legally it didn't happen.

Information on giving a back rub is found later in the chapter, in the skin care section.

Unit 3. Describe guidelines for assisting with grooming

When helping with grooming, always allow residents to do all they can for themselves. Let them make as many choices as possible. Follow the care plan's instructions for what care to give. Some residents may have particular ways of grooming themselves. They may have routines. These routines are important even when people are elderly, sick, or disabled (Fig. 5-15). Remember, some residents may be embarrassed or depressed because they need help with grooming tasks they have done for themselves most of their lives. Be sensitive to this.

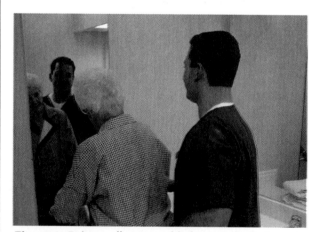

Fig. 5-15. Being well-groomed helps people feel good about themselves.

Nail care should be given if assigned or if nails are dirty or have jagged edges. Never cut a resident's toenails. Poor circulation can lead to infection if skin is accidentally cut while caring for nails. In a diabetic resident, such an infection can lead to a severe wound or even amputation. See chapter 8 for more information on diabetes.

If you are told to give nail care, know what care you are to provide. Never use the same nail equipment on more than one resident.

Providing fingernail care

Equipment: orangewood stick, emery board, lotion, basin, soap, gloves, washcloth, 2 towels, bath thermometer

1. **Wash hands.**
   Provides for infection control.

2. **Identify yourself by name. Identify the resident by name.**
   Resident has right to know identity of his or her caregiver. Addressing resident by name shows respect and establishes correct identification.

3. **Explain procedure to resident. Speak clearly, slowly, and directly. Maintain face-to-face contact whenever possible.**
   Promotes understanding and independence.

4. **Provide for resident's privacy with curtain, screen, or door.**
   Maintains resident's right to privacy and dignity.

5. **If resident is in bed, adjust bed to a safe working level, usually waist high. Lock bed wheels.**
   Prevents injury to you and to resident.

6. **Fill the basin halfway with warm water. Test water temperature with thermometer or your wrist. Ensure it is safe. Water temperature should be 105° F. Have resident check water temperature. Adjust if necessary.**
   Resident's sense of touch may be different than yours; therefore, resident is best able to identify a comfortable water temperature.

7. **Place basin at a comfortable level for resident. Soak the resident's nails in the basin of water. Soak all 10 fingertips for two to four minutes.**
   Nail care is easier if nails are first softened.

8. **Remove hands. Wash hands with soapy washcloth. Rinse. Pat hands dry with towel, including between fingers.**

9. **Put on gloves.**

10. **Place resident's hands on the towel. Use pointed end of the orangewood stick to remove dirt from under the nails (Fig. 5-16).**
    Most pathogens on hands come from beneath the nails.

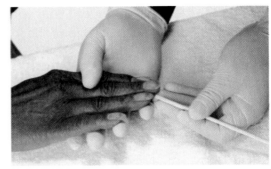

Fig. 5-16.

11. **Wipe orangewood stick on towel after each nail. Wash resident's hands again. Dry them thoroughly.**

12. **Groom nails with file or emery board. File in a curve.**
    Filing in a curve smoothes nails and eliminates edges, which may catch on clothes or tear skin.

13. **Finish with nails smooth and free of rough edges.**

14. **Apply lotion from fingertips to wrists.**

15. **Return bed to appropriate level if previously adjusted.**
    Lowering the bed provides for safety.

16. **Before leaving, place call light within resident's reach.**
    Allows resident to communicate with staff as necessary.

17. **Empty, rinse, and wipe basin. Return to proper storage.**

18. **Dispose of soiled linen in the proper container.**

19. **Remove and dispose of gloves.**

20. **Wash hands.**
    Provides for infection control.

21. **Report any changes in resident to the nurse.**
    Provides nurse with information to assess resident.

22. **Document procedure using facility guidelines.**

    What you write is a legal record of what you did. If you don't document it, legally it didn't happen.

Observing and Reporting Foot Care

- excessive dryness of the skin of the feet
- breaks or tears in the skin
- ingrown nails
- reddened areas on the feet
- drainage or bleeding
- change in color of the skin or nails, especially blackening
- soft, fragile heels
- corns and blisters

Providing foot care

Equipment: basin, bath mat, soap, lotion, gloves, washcloth, 2 towels, bath thermometer, clean socks

Support the foot and ankle throughout procedure.

1. **Wash hands.**

    Provides for infection control.

2. **Identify yourself by name. Identify the resident by name.**

    Resident has right to know identity of his or her caregiver. Addressing resident by name shows respect and establishes correct identification.

3. **Explain procedure to resident. Speak clearly, slowly, and directly. Maintain face-to-face contact whenever possible.**

    Promotes understanding and independence.

4. **Provide for resident's privacy with curtain, screen, or door.**

    Maintains resident's right to privacy and dignity.

5. **If the resident is in bed, adjust bed to a safe working level, usually waist high. Lock bed wheels.**

    Prevents injury to you and to resident.

6. **Fill the basin halfway with warm water. Test water temperature with thermometer or your wrist. Ensure it is safe. Water temperature should be 105° F. Have resident check water temperature. Adjust if necessary.**

    Resident's sense of touch may be different than yours; therefore, resident is best able to identify a comfortable water temperature.

7. **Place basin on the bath mat.**

8. **Remove resident's socks. Completely submerge resident's feet in water. Soak the feet for five to ten minutes.**

9. **Put on gloves.**

10. **Remove one foot from water. Wash entire foot, including between the toes and around nail beds, with soapy washcloth (Fig. 5-17).**

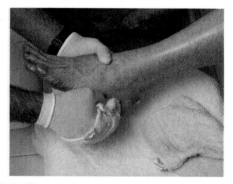

Fig. 5-17.

11. **Rinse entire foot, including between the toes.**

12. **Dry entire foot, including between the toes.**

13. **Repeat steps 10 through 12 for the other foot.**

14. **Put lotion in hand. Warm lotion by rubbing hands together.**

15. **Massage lotion into entire foot (top and bottom), except between the toes, removing excess (if any) with a towel.**

16. **Assist resident to replace socks.**

17. **Return bed to appropriate level if ad-**

justed. **Remove privacy measures.**

Lowering the bed provides for safety.

18. **Empty, rinse, and wipe basin. Return to proper storage.**

19. **Dispose of soiled linen in the proper container.**

20. **Before leaving, place call light within resident's reach.**

Allows resident to communicate with staff as necessary.

21. **Remove and dispose of gloves.**

22. **Wash hands.**

Provides for infection control.

23. **Report any changes in resident to the nurse.**

Provides nurse with information to assess resident.

24. **Document procedure using facility guidelines.**

What you write is a legal record of what you did. If you don't document it, legally it didn't happen.

Handle residents' hair gently. Hair thins as people age. Pieces of hair can be pulled out of the head while combing or brushing it. Also, the skin on residents' heads is fragile. Handle hair carefully.

Pediculosis is an infestation of lice. Lice are tiny bugs that bite into the skin and suck blood to live and grow. Three types of lice are head lice, body lice, and crab or pubic lice. Head lice are usually found on the scalp. Lice are hard to see. Symptoms include itching, bite marks on the scalp, skin sores, and matted, bad-smelling hair and scalp. If you notice any of these symptoms, tell the nurse immediately. They can spread very quickly. Special lice cream, shampoo, or lotion may be used to treat the lice. People who have lice spread it to others. To help prevent the spread of lice, do not share residents' combs, brushes, clothes, wigs, and hats.

Combing or brushing hair

Equipment: comb, brush, towel, mirror, hair care items requested by resident

Use hair care products that the resident prefers for his or her type of hair.

1. **Wash hands.**

Provides for infection control.

2. **Identify yourself by name. Identify the resident by name.**

Resident has right to know identity of his or her caregiver. Addressing resident by name shows respect and establishes correct identification.

3. **Explain procedure to resident. Speak clearly, slowly, and directly. Maintain face-to-face contact whenever possible.**

Promotes understanding and independence.

4. **Provide for resident's privacy with curtain, screen, or door.**

Maintains resident's right to privacy and dignity.

5. **If the bed is adjustable, adjust bed to a safe working level, usually waist high. Lock bed wheels.**

Prevents injury to you and to resident.

6. **Raise head of bed so resident is sitting up. Place a towel under the head or around the shoulders.**

Puts resident in more natural position.

7. **Remove any hair pins, hair ties and clips.**

8. **Remove tangles first by dividing hair into small sections. Gently comb out from ends of hair to scalp.**

Reduces hair breakage, scalp pain and irritation.

9. **After tangles are removed, brush two-inch sections of hair at a time. Brush from roots to ends (Fig. 5-18).**

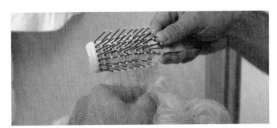

Fig. 5-18.

10. **Style hair as resident prefers. Avoid childish hairstyles. Each resident may prefer different styles and different hair products. Offer mirror to resident.**
Each resident has right to choose. Promotes resident's independence.

11. **Return bed to appropriate position. Remove privacy measures.**
Provides for safety.

12. **Before leaving, place call light within resident's reach.**
Allows resident to communicate with staff as necessary.

13. **Return supplies to proper storage. Clean hair from brush/comb.**

14. **Dispose of soiled linen in the proper container.**

15. **Wash hands.**
Provides for infection control.

16. **Report any changes in resident to nurse.**
Provides nurse with information to assess resident.

17. **Document procedure using facility guidelines.**
What you write is a legal record of what you did. If you don't document it, legally it didn't happen.

Be sure the resident wants you to shave him or help him shave before you begin. Respect personal preferences for shaving. Always wear gloves when shaving a resident. Check with the nurse to know which type of razor the resident uses:

- A **safety razor** has a sharp blade, but with a special safety casing to help prevent cuts. This type of razor requires shaving cream or soap.

- An **electric razor** is the safest and easiest type of razor to use. It does not require soap or shaving cream.

- A **disposable razor** requires shaving cream or soap. It is discarded after use.

Shaving a resident

Equipment: basin, 2 towels, washcloth, bath thermometer, mirror, shaving cream or soap, after-shave, gloves, razor

1. **Wash hands.**
Provides for infection control.

2. **Identify yourself by name. Identify the resident by name.**
Resident has right to know identity of his or her caregiver. Addressing resident by name shows respect and establishes correct identification.

3. **Explain procedure to resident. Speak clearly, slowly, and directly. Maintain face-to-face contact whenever possible.**
Promotes understanding and independence.

4. **Provide for resident's privacy with curtain, screen, or door.**
Maintains resident's right to privacy and dignity.

5. **If bed is adjustable, adjust bed to a safe level, usually waist high. Lock bed wheels.**
Prevents injury to you and to resident.

6. **Raise head of bed so resident is sitting up.**
Puts resident in more natural position.

Shaving using a safety or disposable razor:

7. **Fill bath basin halfway with warm water.**
Hot water opens pores and causes irritation.

8. **Drape towel under resident's chin.**
Protects resident's clothing and bed linen.

9. **Apply gloves.**
Shaving may cause bleeding. Promotes infection control and follows Standard Precautions.

10. **Moisten beard with warm washcloth. Put shaving cream or soap over area.**
Softens skin and hair.

11. **Hold skin taut. Shave beard in downward strokes on face and upward strokes on neck. Rinse razor often in warm water to keep it clean and wet (Fig. 5-19).**
Maximizes hair removal by shaving in the direction of hair growth.

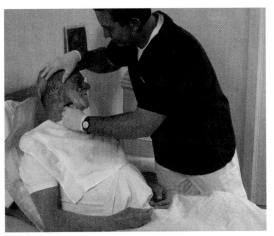

Fig. 5-19.

12. **Offer mirror to resident.**
    Promotes independence.

13. **Wash, rinse, and dry face after the shave. Apply after-shave lotion as requested.**
    Removes soap, which may cause irritation. Improves resident's self-esteem.

14. **Remove towel.**

15. **Remove gloves.**

Shaving using an electric razor:

7. **Do not use an electric razor near any water source, when oxygen is in use, or if resident has a pacemaker.**
   Electricity near water may cause electrocution. Electricity near oxygen may cause an explosion. Electricity near some pacemakers may cause an irregular heartbeat.

8. **Drape towel under resident's chin.**
   Protects resident's clothing and bed linen.

9. **Apply gloves.**
   Shaving may cause bleeding.

10. **Apply pre-shave lotion as resident wishes.**

11. **Hold skin taut. Shave with smooth, even movements (Fig. 5-20). Shave beard with back and forth motion in direction of beard growth with foil shaver. Shave beard in circular motion with three-head shaver.**

12. **Offer mirror to resident.**
    Promotes independence.

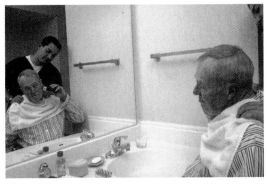

Fig. 5-20.

13. **Apply after-shave lotion as resident wishes.**
    Improves resident's self-esteem.

14. **Remove towel.**

15. **Remove gloves.**

Final steps:

16. **Make sure that resident and environment are free of loose hairs.**

17. **Return bed to appropriate position. Remove privacy measures.**
    Provides for safety.

18. **Before leaving, place call light within resident's reach.**
    Allows resident to communicate with staff as necessary.

19. ***For safety razor*: Rinse safety razor. *For disposable razor*: Dispose of a disposable razor in biohazard container. *For electric razor*: Clean head of electric razor. Remove whiskers from razor. Recap shaving head. Return razor to case.**

20. **Return supplies and equipment to proper storage.**

21. **Wash hands.**
    Provides for infection control.

22. **Report any changes in resident to the nurse.**
    Provides nurse with information to assess resident.

23. **Document procedure using facility guidelines.**
    What you write is a legal record of what you did. If you don't document it, legally it didn't happen.

5

Personal Care Skills

Unit 4. Identify guidelines for good oral hygiene

Oral care, or care of the mouth, teeth, and gums, is done at least twice each day. Oral care should be done after breakfast and after the last meal or snack of the day. It may also be done before a resident eats. Oral care includes brushing teeth and tongue, flossing teeth, and caring for dentures (Fig. 5-21). When giving oral care, wear gloves. Follow Standard Precautions.

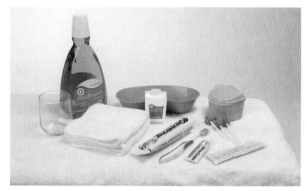

Fig. 5-21. Some supplies needed for oral care.

When you provide oral care, observe the resident's mouth.

Observing and Reporting Oral Care

- irritation
- infection
- raised areas
- coated or swollen tongue
- ulcers, such as canker sores or small, painful, white sores
- flaky, white spots
- dry, cracked, bleeding or chapped lips
- loose, chipped, broken or decayed teeth
- swollen, irritated, bleeding, or whitish gums
- breath that smells bad or fruity
- resident reports of mouth pain

Providing oral care

Equipment: toothbrush, toothpaste, emesis basin, gloves, towel, glass of water

1. **Wash hands.**
   Provides for infection control.

2. **Identify yourself by name. Identify the resident by name.**
   Resident has right to know identity of his or her caregiver. Addressing resident by name shows respect and establishes correct identification.

3. **Explain procedure to resident. Speak clearly, slowly, and directly. Maintain face-to-face contact whenever possible.**
   Promotes understanding and independence.

4. **Provide for resident's privacy with curtain, screen, or door.**
   Maintains resident's right to privacy and dignity.

5. **Adjust bed to a safe working level, usually waist high. Lock bed wheels. Make sure resident is in an upright sitting position.**
   Prevents injury to you and to resident. Prevents fluids from running down resident's throat, causing choking.

6. **Put on gloves.**
   Brushing may cause gums to bleed.

7. **Place towel across resident's chest.**
   Protects resident's clothing and bed linen.

8. **Wet brush. Put on small amount of toothpaste.**
   Water helps distribute toothpaste.

9. **Clean entire mouth (including tongue and all surfaces of teeth). Use gentle strokes. First brush upper teeth, then lower teeth. Use short strokes. Brush back and forth.**
   Brushing upper teeth first minimizes production of saliva in lower part of mouth.

10. **Hold emesis basin to the resident's chin (Fig. 5-22).**

11. **Have resident rinse mouth with water and spit into emesis basin.**
    Removes food particles and toothpaste.

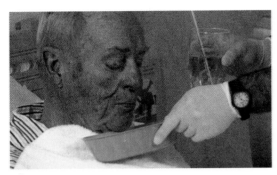

Fig. 5-22.

12. **Wipe resident's mouth and remove towel.**

13. **Dispose of soiled linen in the proper container.**

14. **Clean and return supplies to proper storage.**

15. **Remove gloves. Dispose of gloves properly.**

16. **Return bed to appropriate level. Remove privacy measures.**
Lowering the bed provides for safety.

17. **Before leaving, place call light within resident's reach.**
Allows resident to communicate with staff as necessary.

18. **Wash hands.**
Provides for infection control.

19. **Report any problems with teeth, mouth, tongue, and lips to nurse. This includes odor, cracking, sores, bleeding, and any discoloration.**
Provides nurse with information to assess resident.

20. **Document procedure using facility guidelines.**
What you write is a legal record of what you did. If you don't document it, legally it didn't happen.

👁 *You must brush the tongue when providing oral care.*

Flossing the teeth removes plaque and tartar buildup around the gum line and between the teeth. Teeth may be flossed immediately after or before they are brushed, as the resident prefers. Flossing should not be done for certain residents. Follow the care plan.

Flossing teeth

Equipment: floss, cup with water, emesis basin, gloves, towel

1. **Wash hands.**
Provides for infection control.

2. **Identify yourself by name. Identify the resident by name.**
Resident has right to know identity of his or her caregiver. Addressing resident by name shows respect and establishes correct identification.

3. **Explain procedure to resident. Speak clearly, slowly, and directly. Maintain face-to-face contact whenever possible.**
Promotes understanding and independence.

4. **Provide for resident's privacy with curtain, screen, or door.**
Maintains resident's right to privacy and dignity.

5. **Adjust the bed to a safe level. Lock bed wheels. Make sure the resident is in an upright sitting position.**
Prevents injury to you and to resident. Prevents fluids from running down resident's throat, causing choking.

6. **Put on gloves.**
Flossing may cause gums to bleed.

7. **Wrap the ends of floss securely around each index finger (Fig. 5-23).**

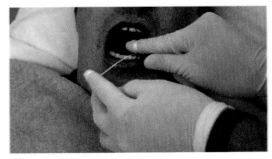

Fig. 5-23.

8. **Starting with the back teeth, place floss between teeth. Move it down the surface of the tooth. Use a gentle sawing motion (Fig. 5-24).**
Being gentle protects gums.

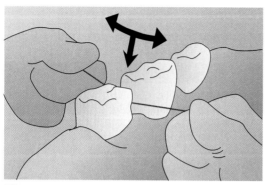

Fig. 5-24.

Continue to the gum line. At the gum line, curve the floss into a letter C. Slip it gently into the space between the gum and tooth. Then go back up, scraping that side of the tooth (Fig. 5-25). Repeat this on the side of the other tooth.

Removes food and prevents tooth decay.

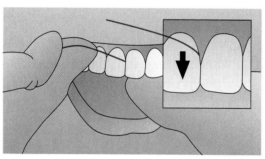

Fig. 5-25.

9. After every two teeth, unwind floss from your fingers. Move it so you are using a clean area. Floss all teeth.

10. Offer water to rinse the mouth. Ask the resident to spit it into the basin.
Flossing loosens food. Rinsing removes it.

11. Offer resident a face towel when done flossing all teeth.
Promotes dignity.

12. Dispose of soiled linen in the proper container.

13. Clean and return supplies to proper storage.

14. Remove and dispose of gloves properly.

15. Return bed to appropriate position.

Remove privacy measures.
Lowering the bed provides for safety.

16. Before leaving, place call light within resident's reach.
Allows resident to communicate with staff as necessary.

17. Wash hands.
Provides for infection control.

18. Report any problems with teeth, mouth, tongue, and lips to nurse. This includes odor, cracking, sores, bleeding, and any discoloration.
Provides nurse with information to assess resident.

19. Document procedure using facility guidelines.
What you write is a legal record of what you did. If you don't document it, legally it didn't happen.

Dentures are artificial teeth. They are expensive. Take good care of them. Handle dentures carefully to avoid breaking or chipping them. If a resident's dentures break, he or she cannot eat. When cleaning dentures, wear gloves. Notify the nurse if a resident's dentures do not fit properly, are chipped, or are missing.

When storing dentures, place them in a denture cup with the resident's name on it. Store in solution or cool water. Make sure to match the dentures to the correct resident.

Cleaning and storing dentures

Equipment: denture brush or toothbrush, denture cleanser or tablet, labeled denture cup, 2 towels, gloves

1. Wash hands.
Provides for infection control.

2. Put on gloves.
Prevents you from coming into contact with body fluids.

3. Line sink/basin with a towel(s) or fill sink with water.
Prevents dentures from breaking if dropped.

4. Rinse dentures in cool running water before brushing them. Do not use hot water.

Hot water may damage dentures.

5. Apply toothpaste or cleanser to toothbrush.

6. Brush the dentures on all surfaces (Fig. 5-26).

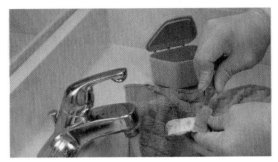

Fig. 5-26.

7. Rinse all surfaces of dentures under cool running water. Do not use hot water.

Hot water may damage dentures.

8. Rinse denture cup before placing clean dentures in it.

Removes pathogens.

9. Place dentures in clean denture cup with solution or cool water (Fig. 5-27). Make sure cup is labeled with resident's name. Return denture cup to storage.

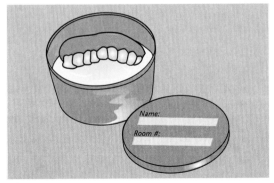

Fig. 5-27.

10. Clean and return the equipment to proper storage.

11. Dispose of towels in appropriate container or drain sink.

12. Remove and dispose of gloves properly.

13. Wash hands.

Provides for infection control.

14. Report any changes in appearance of dentures to the nurse.

Provides nurse with information to assess resident.

15. Document procedure using facility guidelines.

What you write is a legal record of what you did. If you don't document it, legally it didn't happen.

Although residents who are unconscious cannot eat, breathing through the mouth causes saliva to dry in the mouth. Good mouth care needs to be performed more frequently to keep the mouth clean and moist. Swabs with a mixture of lemon juice and glycerine are sometimes used to soothe the gums. But these may further dry the gums if used too often. Follow the care plan regarding the use of swabs.

With unconscious residents, use as little liquid as possible when giving oral care. Because the person's swallowing reflex is weak, he or she is at risk for aspiration. **Aspiration** is the inhalation of food or drink into the lungs. Aspiration can cause pneumonia or death. Turning unconscious residents on their sides before giving oral care can also help prevent aspiration. Chapter 7 has more information on aspiration.

Providing oral care for the unconscious resident

Equipment: sponge swabs, padded tongue blade, towel, emesis basin, gloves, lip moisturizer, cleaning solution (check the care plan)

1. Wash hands.

Provides for infection control.

2. Identify yourself by name. Identify the resident by name. Even residents who are unconscious may be able to hear

5

Personal Care Skills

you. Always speak to them as you would to any resident.

Resident has right to know identity of his or her caregiver. Addressing resident by name shows respect and establishes correct identification.

3. Explain procedure to resident. Speak clearly, slowly, and directly. Maintain face-to-face contact whenever possible.

Promotes understanding. The resident may be able to hear and understand even though he is unconscious.

4. Provide for resident's privacy with curtain, screen, or door.

Maintains resident's right to privacy and dignity.

5. Adjust bed to a safe level, usually waist high. Lock bed wheels.

Prevents injury to you and to resident.

6. Put on gloves.

Protects you from coming into contact with body fluids.

7. Turn resident's head to the side. Place a towel under his cheek and chin. Place an emesis basin next to the cheek and chin for excess fluid.

Protects resident's clothing and bed linen.

8. Hold mouth open with padded tongue blade.

Enables you to safely clean mouth.

9. Dip swab in cleaning solution. Wipe teeth, gums, tongue, and inside surfaces of mouth. Change swab often. Repeat until the mouth is clean (Fig. 5-28).

Stimulates gums and removes mucus.

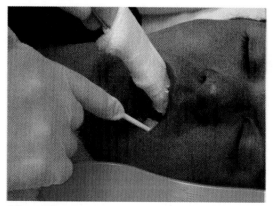

Fig. 5-28.

10. Rinse with clean swab dipped in water.

Removes solution from mouth.

11. Remove the towel and basin. Pat lips or face dry if needed. Apply lip moisturizer.

Prevents lips from drying and cracking. Improves resident's comfort.

12. Dispose of soiled linen in the proper container.

13. Clean and return supplies to proper storage.

14. Remove and dispose of gloves properly.

15. Return bed to appropriate position. Remove privacy measures.

Lowering the bed provides for safety.

16. Before leaving, place call light within resident's reach.

Allows resident to communicate with staff as necessary.

17. Wash hands.

Provides for infection control.

18. Report any changes in resident to the nurse.

Provides nurse with information to assess resident.

19. Document procedure using facility guidelines.

What you write is a legal record of what you did. If you don't document it, legally it didn't happen.

Unit 5. List guidelines for assisting with dressing

When helping a resident with dressing, know what limitations he or she has. If he or she has a weakened side from a stroke or injury, that side is called the **affected side**. It will be weaker. Never refer to the weaker side as the "bad side," or talk about the "bad" leg or arm. Use the terms **weaker** or **involved** to refer to the affected side. The weaker arm is usually placed through a sleeve first (Fig. 5-29). When a leg is weak, it is easier if the resident sits down to pull the pants over both legs.

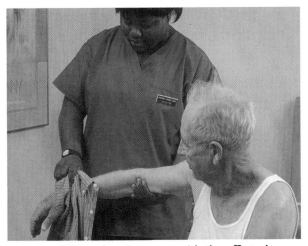

Fig. 5-29. When dressing, start with the affected (weaker) side first.

Residents should do as much for themselves as they can when dressing. This includes choosing the clothes they will wear. This encourages independence and promotes self-care.

Guidelines
Helping a Resident Dress and Undress

- The resident's preferences should be asked and followed.

- Let the resident choose clothing for the day. Check to see if it is clean, appropriate for the weather, and in good condition. Encourage the resident to dress in regular clothes rather than nightclothes.

- The resident should do as much to dress or undress himself as possible.

- Provide privacy.

- Roll or fold stockings or socks down when putting them on. Slip over the toes and foot, then unroll into place.

- Front-fastening bras are easier for residents to manage by themselves. Bras that fasten in back can be put around the waist and fastened first. Then rotate around and move bra up.

- Place the weaker arm or leg through the garment first, then the stronger arm. When undressing, do the opposite.

Dressing a resident with an affected (weak) right arm

Equipment: clean clothes of resident's choice, non-skid footwear

When putting on all items, move resident's body gently and naturally. Avoid force and over-extension of limbs and joints.

1. **Wash hands.**
   Provides for infection control.

2. **Identify yourself by name. Identify the resident by name.**
   Resident has right to know identity of his or her caregiver. Addressing resident by name shows respect and establishes correct identification.

3. **Explain procedure to resident. Speak clearly, slowly, and directly. Maintain face-to-face contact whenever possible.**
   Promotes understanding and independence.

4. **Provide for resident's privacy with curtain, screen, or door.**
   Maintains resident's right to privacy and dignity.

5. **Ask resident what she would like to wear. Dress her in outfit of choice (Fig. 5-30).**
   Promotes resident's right to choose.

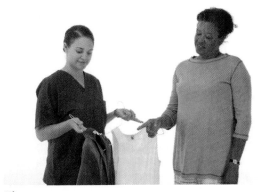

Fig. 5-30.

6. **Remove resident's gown. Do not completely expose resident. Take off stronger side first when undressing.**
   Maintains resident's dignity and right to privacy by not exposing body.

7. **Assist resident to put the right (affected/weak) arm through the right**

sleeve of the shirt, sweater, or slip before placing garment on left (unaffected) arm.

Dressing affected side first requires less movement and reduces stress to joints.

8. **Help resident to put on skirt, pants, or dress.**

9. **Place bed at a safe level for resident, usually the lowest position.**

10. **Apply non-skid footwear. Tie laces.**
    Promotes resident's safety.

11. **Finish with resident dressed appropriately. Make sure clothing is right-side-out and zippers/buttons are fastened.**

12. **Remove privacy measures. Place gown in soiled linen container.**

13. **Before leaving, place call light within resident's reach.**
    Allows resident to communicate with staff as necessary.

14. **Wash hands.**
    Provides for infection control.

15. **Report any changes in resident to the nurse.**
    Provides nurse with information to assess resident.

16. **Document procedure using facility guidelines.**
    What you write is a legal record of what you did. If you don't document it, legally it didn't happen.

👁 *Always dress a resident's weaker side first.*

IV stands for **intravenous**, or into a vein. Medication, nutrition, or fluids drip from a bag suspended on a pole or are pumped by a portable pump through a tube and into the vein. Chapter 6 has more information on IVs.

Guidelines
Dressing a Resident with an IV

Dressing and undressing residents with IVs requires special care.

- Never disconnect IV lines or turn off the pump. The nurse will be responsible for unhooking IV tubing from the pump.

- Remove or assist in removing clothing from the side without the IV. Then hold garment while undressing side with IV.

- Slide clothing over the tubing. Lift the IV bag off the hook and pull the gown over the bag.

- Always keep bag above IV site on body.

- Apply clean clothing first to side with the IV. Slide the correct arm opening over the bag, then over the tubing and the resident's IV arm.

🏳 *Choice of what to wear is part of a person's identity; it is a very personal decision. This remains true even when a person is elderly, ill, or disabled. Handle residents' clothing carefully. Treat religious or spiritual items of clothing with respect.*

Unit 6. Explain guidelines for assisting with toileting

Residents who are unable to get out of bed to go to the bathroom may be given a bedpan, a urinal, or a fracture pan. A **fracture pan** is a bedpan that is flatter than the regular bedpan. It is used for residents who cannot assist with raising their hips onto a regular bedpan (Fig. 5-31).

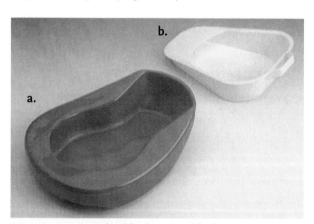

Fig. 5-31. a) Standard bedpan and b) fracture pan.

Women will use a bedpan for urination and bowel movements. Men will generally use a urinal for urination and a bedpan for bowel movements (Fig. 5-32). If facility policy, rinse this equipment with an approved disinfectant after each use. It is usually kept in the bathroom or bottom drawer of nightstand between uses. Residents who share bathrooms may need to have urinals and bedpans labeled. Never place this equipment on an overbed table or on top of a side table.

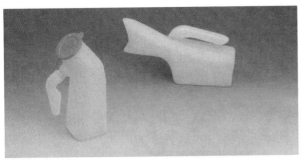

Fig. 5-32. Urinals.

Residents who are able to get out of bed but cannot walk to the bathroom may use a portable commode. A **portable commode** is a chair with a toilet seat and a removable container underneath (Fig. 5-33).

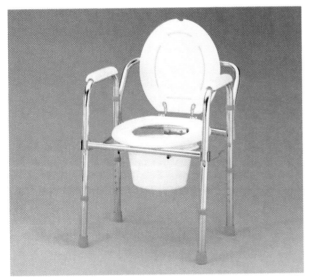

Fig. 5-33. A portable commode. (Photo courtesy of Nova Ortho Med, Inc.)

Wastes such as urine and feces can carry infection. Always dispose of wastes in the toilet. Be careful not to spill or splash. Wear gloves when handling bedpans, urinals, or basins that contain wastes. This includes dirty bath water. Wash these containers thoroughly with an approved disinfectant. Rinse and dry. Return to storage.

Assisting resident with use of bedpan

Equipment: bedpan, bedpan cover, protective pad or sheet, bath blanket, toilet paper, washcloths or wipes, 2 pairs of gloves

1. **Wash hands.**
   Provides for infection control.

2. **Identify yourself by name. Identify the resident by name.**
   Resident has right to know identity of his or her caregiver. Addressing resident by name shows respect and establishes correct identification.

3. **Explain procedure to resident. Speak clearly, slowly, and directly. Maintain face-to-face contact whenever possible.**
   Promotes understanding and independence.

4. **Provide for resident's privacy with curtain, screen, or door.**
   Maintains resident's right to privacy and dignity.

5. **Before placing bedpan, lower head of bed. Lock bed wheels.**
   When bed is flat, resident can be moved without working against gravity.

6. **Apply gloves.**
   Prevents contact with body fluids.

7. **Cover the resident with a bath blanket. Ask him to hold it while you pull down the top covers underneath. Do not expose more of him than you have to.**
   Maintains resident's right to privacy and dignity.

8. **Place a protective pad under the resident's buttocks and hips. To do this, have the resident roll toward you. If the resident cannot do this, you must turn him toward you (see later in this chapter). Be sure resident cannot roll off the bed. Move to empty side of bed. Place protective sheet on the area where the**

resident will lie on his back. The side of protective sheet nearest the resident should be fanfolded (folded several times into pleats). Ask resident to roll onto his back, or roll him as you did before. Unfold rest of protective sheet so it completely covers area under and around the resident's hips. (Fig. 5-34)

Prevents linen from being soiled.

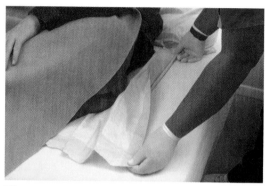

Fig. 5-34.

9. Ask resident to remove undergarments or help him do so.

   Promotes independence.

10. If resident is able, ask him to raise hips by pushing with feet and hands. Place bedpan correctly under resident's buttocks (Standard bedpan: Position bedpan so wider end of pan is aligned with resident's buttocks (Fig. 5-35); Fracture pan: Position bedpan with handle toward foot of bed). If a resident cannot help you in any way, keep the bed flat and roll the resident onto the far side. Slip the bedpan under the hips and roll him back onto the bedpan.

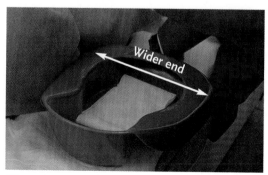

Fig. 5-35.

11. Raise head of bed after placing bedpan under resident.

    Puts resident in comfortable position for voiding.

12. Put toilet tissue within resident's reach.

13. Leave call light within resident's reach while resident is using bedpan. Ask resident to signal when finished.

    Ensures ability to communicate need for assistance.

14. Without removing gloves, remain outside the room until called by the resident. When called, return and lower head of bed.

    Places resident in proper position to remove pan.

15. Remove bedpan carefully. Cover bedpan.

    Promotes infection control and odor control. Provides dignity for resident.

16. Provide perineal care if assistance is needed. Remember to wipe female residents from front to back.

    Prevents spread of pathogens, which may cause urinary tract infection.

17. Empty contents of bedpan into toilet. Note color, odor, and consistency of contents.

    Changes may be first sign of medical problem.

18. Rinse bedpan. Pour rinse water into toilet. Use approved disinfectant if facility policy.

19. Remove and dispose of gloves properly.

20. Wash hands.

    Provides for infection control.

21. Put on clean gloves.

    Prevents contact with body fluids.

22. Return bedpan to proper storage.

23. Assist resident to wash hands after using bedpan. Dispose of soiled washcloth or wipes in proper container. Help resident put on undergarment.

    Handwashing is the best way to prevent the spread of infection.

24. Remove and dispose of gloves properly.

25. Return bed to appropriate position.

Remove privacy measures.
Lowering the bed provides for resident's safety.

26. **Before leaving, place call light within resident's reach.**
Allows resident to communicate with staff as necessary.

27. **Wash hands.**
Provides for infection control.

28. **Report any changes in resident to the nurse.**
Provides nurse with information to assess resident.

29. **Document procedure using facility guidelines.**
What you write is a legal record of what you did. If you don't document it, legally it didn't happen.

👁 *Remember to position a standard bedpan so that the wider end is aligned with a resident's buttocks. A fracture pan should be positioned with the handle toward the foot of the bed.*

Assisting a male resident with a urinal

Equipment: urinal, protective pad or sheet, washcloths or wipes, gloves

1. **Wash hands.**
Provides for infection control.

2. **Identify yourself by name. Identify the resident by name.**
Resident has right to know identity of his or her caregiver. Addressing resident by name shows respect and establishes correct identification.

3. **Explain procedure to resident. Speak clearly, slowly, and directly. Maintain face-to-face contact whenever possible.**
Promotes understanding and independence.

4. **Provide for resident's privacy with curtain, screen, or door.**
Maintains resident's right to privacy and dignity.

5. **Lock bed wheels. Apply gloves.**
Prevents injury. Prevents you from coming into contact with body fluids.

6. **Place a protective pad under the resident's buttocks and hips.**
Prevents linen from being soiled.

7. **Hand the urinal to the resident. If the resident cannot do so himself, place urinal between his legs and position penis inside the urinal (Fig. 5-36). Replace bed covers.**
Promotes independence, dignity and privacy.

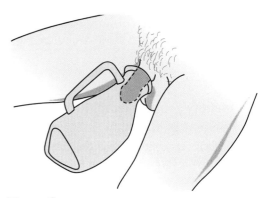

Fig. 5-36.

8. **Leave call light within resident's reach while resident is using urinal. Ask resident to signal when finished.**
Ensures ability to communicate need for assistance.

9. **Remove urinal. Empty contents into toilet. Note color, odor, and qualities (e.g. cloudy) of contents.**
Changes may be first sign of medical problem.

10. **Rinse urinal. Pour rinse water into toilet. Use approved disinfectant if facility policy. Return to proper storage.**

11. **Remove and dispose of gloves.**

12. **Assist resident to wash hands after using urinal. Dispose of soiled washcloth or wipes properly.**
Handwashing is the best way to prevent the spread of infection.

13. **Before leaving, place call light within resident's reach.**
Allows resident to communicate with staff as necessary.

14. **Wash hands.**
Provides for infection control.

15. **Report any changes in resident to the nurse.**
Provides nurse with information to assess resident.

5

Personal Care Skills

16. **Document procedure using facility guidelines.**

    What you write is a legal record of what you did. If you don't document it, legally it didn't happen.

Helping a resident use a portable commode

Equipment: portable commode with basin, toilet paper, washcloths or wipes, gloves

1. **Wash hands.**

   Provides for infection control.

2. **Identify yourself by name. Identify the resident by name.**

   Resident has right to know identity of his or her caregiver. Addressing resident by name shows respect and establishes correct identification.

3. **Explain procedure to resident. Speak clearly, slowly, and directly. Maintain face-to-face contact whenever possible.**

   Promotes understanding and independence.

4. **Provide for resident's privacy with curtain, screen, or door.**

   Maintains resident's right to privacy and dignity.

5. **Help resident out of bed and to portable commode. Make sure resident is wearing non-skid shoes.**

6. **If needed, help resident remove clothing and sit comfortably on toilet seat. Put toilet tissue within reach.**

7. **Leave call light within reach while resident is using commode. Ask resident to signal when done.**

   Ensures ability to communicate need for assistance.

8. **Return and apply gloves.**

   Prevents you from coming into contact with body fluids.

9. **Give perineal care if help is needed. Wipe female residents from front to back.**

   Prevents spread of pathogens, which may cause urinary tract infection.

10. **Assist resident to wash hands after using commode. Dispose of soiled washcloth or wipes properly.**

    Handwashing is the best way to prevent the spread of infection.

11. **Assist back to bed.**

12. **Remove waste container. Empty into toilet. Note color, odor, and consistency of contents.**

    Changes may be first sign of medical problem.

13. **Rinse container. Pour rinse water into toilet. Use approved disinfectant if facility policy. Return to proper storage.**

14. **Remove and dispose of gloves properly.**

15. **Before leaving, place call light within resident's reach.**

    Allows resident to communicate with staff as necessary.

16. **Wash hands.**

    Provides for infection control.

17. **Report any changes in resident to the nurse.**

    Provides nurse with information to assess resident.

18. **Document procedure using facility guidelines.**

    What you write is a legal record of what you did. If you don't document it, legally it didn't happen.

Some people cannot control the muscles of the bowels or bladder. They are said to be **incontinent**. This is not a normal part of aging. Incontinence can occur in residents who are confined to bed, ill, paralyzed, or who have circulatory or nervous system diseases or injuries. Diarrhea can also cause temporary incontinence.

Residents who are incontinent need reassurance and understanding. Be caring and empathetic. Offer them a bedpan or take them to the bathroom more frequently. Keep them clean, dry, and free from odor. Some residents will wear disposable incontinence pads or briefs for adults. Change wet briefs immediately. Residents who are incontinent will need good skin care. Urine and feces are very irritating to the skin. They should be washed off completely by bathing and good perineal care.

Urinary incontinence is also a major risk factor for pressure sores. Rules for documenting incontinence have changed. The new MDS counts any time a resident's skin or anything touching a resident's skin (pad, brief, or underwear) is wet from urine as an episode of incontinence. This is true even if it is a small amount of urine. This is important to help prevent pressure sores.

The survey team will look to see that each resident's elimination needs are met. This includes a toileting schedule to lessen episodes of incontinence.

Providing perineal care for an incontinent resident

Equipment: 2 clean protective pads, 4 washcloths or wipes, 1 towel, gloves, basin with warm water, soap, bath blanket, bath thermometer

1. **Wash hands.**
   Provides for infection control.

2. **Identify yourself by name. Identify the resident by name.**
   Resident has right to know identity of his or her caregiver. Addressing resident by name shows respect and establishes correct identification.

3. **Explain procedure to resident. Speak clearly, slowly, and directly. Maintain face-to-face contact whenever possible.**
   Promotes understanding and independence.

4. **Provide for resident's privacy with curtain, screen, or door.**
   Maintains resident's right to privacy and dignity.

5. **Adjust bed to a safe working level, usually waist high. Lock bed wheels.**
   Prevents injury to you and to resident.

6. **Lower head of bed. Position resident lying flat on his or her back. Raise the**
side rail farthest from you.

7. **Test water temperature with thermometer or your wrist. Ensure it is safe. Water temperature should be 105° to 109° F. Have resident check water temperature. Adjust if necessary.**
   Resident's sense of touch may be different than yours; therefore, resident is best able to identify a comfortable water temperature.

8. **Put on gloves.**
   Prevents you from coming into contact with body fluids.

9. **Cover resident with bath blanket. Move top linens to foot of bed.**
   Maintains resident's right to privacy and dignity.

10. **Remove soiled protective pad from underneath resident by turning resident on his side, away from you. (See procedure *Turning a Resident* later in this chapter.) Roll soiled pad into itself with wet side in/dry side out.**
    Keeps linen from getting wet.

11. **Place clean protective pad under his or her buttocks.**
    Keeps linen from getting wet.

12. **Return resident to lying on his back.**

13. **Expose perineal area only. Clean perineal area.**

    For a female resident: Wash the perineum with soap and water from *front to back*. Use single strokes. Do not wash from the back to the front. This may cause infection. Use a clean area of washcloth or clean washcloth for each stroke. First wipe the center of the perineum, then each side. Spread the labia majora, the outside folds of perineal skin that protect the urinary meatus and the vaginal opening. Wipe from front to back on each side. Rinse the area in the same way. Dry entire perineal area. Move from front to back, using a blotting motion with towel. Ask resident to turn on her side. Wash, rinse, and dry

5

Personal Care Skills

5

Personal Care Skills

buttocks and anal area. Cleanse the anal area without contaminating the perineal area.

For a male resident: If the resident is uncircumcised, retract the foreskin. Gently push skin towards the base of penis.

Hold the penis by the shaft. Wash in a circular motion from the tip down to the base. Use a clean area of washcloth or clean washcloth for each stroke. Rinse the penis. If resident is uncircumcised, gently return foreskin to normal position. Then wash the scrotum and groin. The groin is the area from the pubis to the upper thighs. Rinse and pat dry. Ask the resident to turn on his side. Wash, rinse, and dry buttocks and anal area. Cleanse the anal area without contaminating the perineal area.

14. **Turn resident on his side away from you. Remove the wet protective pad after drying buttocks.**

15. **Place a dry protective pad under the resident.**
    Keeps linen from getting wet.

16. **Reposition the resident.**

17. **Replace top covers. Remove bath blanket.**

18. **Place soiled linens, clothing and protective pad in proper containers.**

19. **Empty, rinse, and wipe basin. Return to proper storage.**

20. **Remove and dispose of gloves properly.**

21. **Return bed to appropriate level. Remove privacy measures.**
    Lowering the bed provides for safety.

22. **Put call light within resident's reach.**
    Allows resident to communicate with staff as necessary.

23. **Wash hands.**
    Provides for infection control.

24. **Report any changes in resident to the nurse.**
    Provides nurse with information to assess resident.

25. **Document procedure using facility guidelines.**
    What you write is a legal record of what you did. If you don't document it, legally it didn't happen.

👁 *When washing perineal area, use a clean area of the washcloth or clean washcloth for each stroke.*

Constipation is the difficult and often painful elimination of a hard, dry stool. Constipation occurs when the feces move too slowly through the intestine. This can result from decreased fluid intake, poor diet, inactivity, medications, aging, disease, or ignoring the need to eliminate. Signs of constipation include abdominal swelling, gas, irritability, and record of no recent bowel movement.

Treatment often includes increasing the amount of fiber eaten, increasing fluid intake and activity level, and possibly medication. An enema or suppository may be ordered. An **enema** is a specific amount of water flowed into the colon to eliminate stool. A **suppository** is a medication given rectally to cause a bowel movement. If allowed and trained to do so, follow facility policy on assisting with these treatments.

A **fecal impaction** results from unrelieved constipation. It is a hard stool stuck in the rectum. It cannot be expelled. Symptoms include no stool for several days and oozing of liquid stool. Cramping, abdominal swelling, vomiting, and rectal pain also occur. When an impaction occurs, a healthcare provider will insert one or two gloved fingers into the rectum and break the mass into fragments. Then it can be passed.

Unit 7. Identify guidelines for good skin care

Immobility reduces the amount of blood that circulates to the skin. Residents who have less mobility have more risk of skin deterioration at pressure points. **Pressure points** are areas of the body that bear much of its weight. Pressure points are mainly located at bony prominences. **Bony prominences** are areas of the body where the bone lies close to the skin. These areas include elbows, shoulder blades, tailbone, hip bones, ankles, heels, and the back of the neck and head. The skin here is at a much higher risk for skin breakdown.

Other areas at risk are the ears, the area under the breasts, and the scrotum (Fig. 5-37). The pressure on these areas reduces circulation, decreasing the amount of oxygen the cells receive. Warmth and moisture also add to skin breakdown. Once the surface of the skin is weakened, pathogens can invade and cause infection. When infection occurs, the healing process slows down.

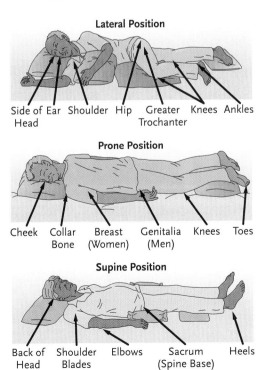

Fig. 5-37. Pressure sore danger zones.

When skin begins to break down, it becomes pale, white, or a reddened color. Darker skin may look purple. The resident may also feel tingling or burning in the area. This discoloration does not go away, even when the resident's position is changed. If pressure is allowed to continue, the area will further deteriorate, or break down. The resulting wound is called a **pressure sore**, pressure ulcer, bed sore, or decubitus ulcer.

Once a pressure sore forms, it can get bigger, deeper, and infected. Most pressure sores develop within a few weeks of admission to a nursing home. Pressure sores are painful and difficult to heal. They can lead to life-threatening infection. Prevention is very important.

There are four accepted stages of pressure sores (Fig. 5-38):

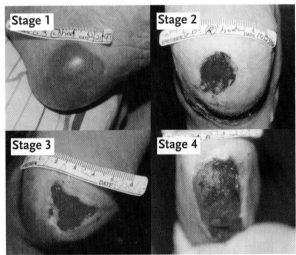

Fig. 5-38. Pressure sores are categorized by four stages. (Photos courtesy of Dr. Tamara D. Fishman and The Wound Care Institute, Inc.)

- **Stage 1**: Area where skin is intact but there is redness that is not relieved within 15 to 30 minutes after removing pressure.

- **Stage 2**: Partial skin loss involving the outer and/or inner layer of skin. The ulcer is superficial. It looks like a blister or a shallow crater.

- **Stage 3**: Full skin loss involving damage or death of tissue that may extend down to but not through the tissue that covers muscle. The ulcer looks like a deep crater.

- **Stage 4**: Full skin loss with major destruction, tissue death, damage to muscle, bone, or supporting structures.

Observing and Reporting Resident's Skin

Report any of these to the nurse:

- pale, white or reddened, or purple areas, blisters or bruises on the skin

- complaints of tingling, warmth, or burning of the skin

- dry or flaking skin

- itching or scratching

- rash or any skin discoloration

- swelling

- blisters

- fluid or blood draining from skin

- broken skin

- wounds or ulcers on the skin

- changes in wound or ulcer (size, depth, drainage, color, odor)

- redness or broken skin between toes or around toenails

In ebony complexions, also look for

- any change in the feel of the tissue, any change in the appearance of the skin, such as the "orange-peel" look, a purplish hue, and extremely dry, crust-like areas that might be covering a tissue break upon a closer look

Guidelines
Basic Skin Care

- Report changes in a resident's skin.

- Provide regular care for skin to keep it clean and dry. When complete baths are not given or taken every day, check the resident's skin and provide skin care daily.

- Reposition immobile residents at least every two hours.

- Give frequent and thorough skin care as often as needed for incontinent residents. Change clothing and linens often as well. Check on them every two hours or as needed.

- Do not scratch or irritate the skin in any way. Report to the nurse if a resident wears shoes or slippers that cause blisters or sores.

- Massage the skin often. Use light, circular strokes to increase circulation. Use little or no pressure on bony areas.

- Do not massage a white, red, or purple area or put any pressure on it. Massage the healthy skin and tissue around the area.

- Be careful during transfers. Avoid pulling or tearing fragile skin.

For residents who are not mobile or cannot change positions easily, remember:

- Keep the bottom sheet tight and free from wrinkles. Keep the bed free from crumbs.

- Do not pull the resident across sheets during transfers or repositioning. This causes shearing, or pressure or friction, when the surfaces rub against each other.

- Place a sheepskin, chamois skin, or bed pad under the back and buttocks to absorb moisture or perspiration that may build up and to protect the skin from irritating bed linens.

- Relieve pressure under bony prominences. Place foam rubber or sheepskin pads under them. Heel and elbow protectors made of foam and sheepskin are available (Fig. 5-39).

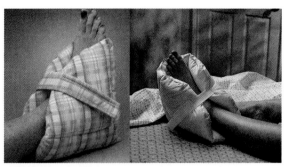

Fig. 5-39. Heel protectors. (Reprinted with permission of Briggs Corporation, 800-247-2343.)

- A bed or chair can be made softer with flotation pads.

- Residents in chairs or wheelchairs need to be repositioned often, too. Reposition residents every 15 minutes if they are in a wheelchair or chair and cannot change positions easily.

Many positioning devices are available to help make residents more comfortable and safe.

Guidelines
Using Positioning Devices

- Backrests can be regular pillows or special wedge-shaped foam pillows.

- Bed cradles are used to keep the bed covers from pushing down on resident's feet.

- Use **draw sheets**, or turning sheets, under residents who cannot help with turning in bed, lifting, or moving up in bed. Draw sheets help prevent skin damage caused by shearing.

- Footboards are padded boards placed against the resident's feet to keep them flexed (Fig. 5-40).

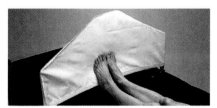

Fig. 5-40. Footboards help prevent pressure sores. (Reprinted with permission of Briggs Corporation, 800-247-2343.)

- Hand rolls keep the fingers from curling tightly (Fig. 5-41).

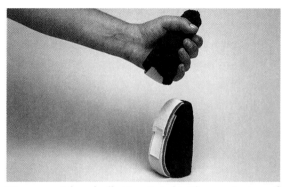

Fig. 5-41. A handroll. (Reprinted with permission of Briggs Corporation, 800-247-2343.)

- Splints may be prescribed by a doctor to keep a resident's joints in the correct position.

The survey team will look to see that staff have taken all necessary steps to prevent pressure sores. This includes turning and positioning residents, helping residents with eating and drinking, and managing episodes of incontinence.

A back rub can help relax your resident. It can make him more comfortable and increase circulation. Back rubs are often given after baths.

Giving a back rub

Equipment: cotton blanket or towel, lotion

1. **Wash hands.**
   Provides for infection control.

2. **Identify yourself by name. Identify the resident by name.**
   Resident has right to know identity of his or her caregiver. Addressing resident by name shows respect and establishes correct identification.

3. **Explain procedure to resident. Speak clearly, slowly, and directly. Maintain face-to-face contact whenever possible.**
   Promotes understanding and independence.

4. **Provide for resident's privacy with curtain, screen, or door.**
   Maintains resident's right to privacy and dignity.

5

Personal Care Skills

5. **Adjust bed to a safe working level, usually waist high. Lock bed wheels.**
    Prevents injury to you and to resident.

6. **Position resident lying on his side or his stomach. Many elderly residents find lying on their stomachs uncomfortable. If so, put him on his side. Cover with a cotton blanket. Expose back to the top of the buttocks. Back rubs can also be given with the resident sitting up.**

7. **Warm lotion by putting bottle in warm water for five minutes. Run your hands under warm water. Pour lotion on your hands. Rub them together. Always put lotion on your hands rather than directly on resident's skin.**
    Increases resident's comfort.

8. **Place hands on each side of upper part of the buttocks. Use the full palm of hand. Make long, smooth upward strokes with both hands. Move along each side of the spine, up to the shoulders (Figs. 5-42 and 5-43). Circle hands outward. Move back along outer edges of the back. At buttocks, make another circle. Move hands back up to the shoulders. Without taking hands from resident's skin, repeat this motion for three to five minutes.**
    Long upward strokes release muscle tension; circular strokes increase circulation in muscle areas.

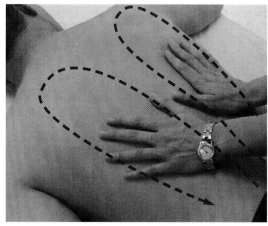

Fig. 5-43. A resident on his stomach.

9. **Knead with the first two fingers and thumb of each hand. Place them at base of the spine. Move upward together along each side of the spine. Apply gentle downward pressure with fingers and thumbs. Follow same direction as with the long smooth strokes, circling at shoulders and buttocks.**

10. **Gently massage bony areas (spine, shoulder blades, hip bones). Use circular motions of fingertips. If any of these areas are red, massage around them rather than on them.**
    Redness indicates that skin is already irritated and fragile.

11. **Finish with some long, smooth strokes.**

12. **Dry the back if extra lotion remains on it.**

13. **Help the resident with getting dressed.**

14. **Remove blanket.**

15. **Store supplies. Place soiled clothing and linens in proper containers.**

16. **Return bed to proper position. Remove privacy measures.**
    Provides for resident's safety.

17. **Before leaving, place call light within resident's reach.**
    Allows resident to communicate with staff as necessary.

18. **Wash hands.**
    Provides for infection control.

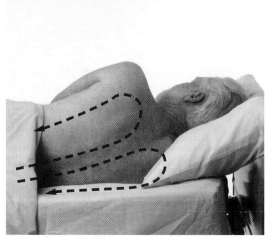

Fig. 5-42. A resident on his side.

19. **Report any changes in resident to the nurse.**

    Provides nurse with information to assess resident.

20. **Document procedure using facility guidelines.**

    What you write is a legal record of what you did. If you don't document it, legally it didn't happen.

Unit 8. Explain the guidelines for safely positioning and transferring residents

Positioning means helping residents into positions that will be comfortable and healthy for them. Bedbound residents should be repositioned at least every two hours. Follow the care plan. Always check the skin for signs of irritation whenever you reposition a resident.

Assisting resident to move up in bed

1. **Wash hands.**

    Provides for infection control.

2. **Identify yourself by name. Identify the resident by name.**

    Resident has right to know identity of his or her caregiver. Addressing resident by name shows respect and establishes correct identification.

3. **Explain procedure to resident. Speak clearly, slowly, and directly. Maintain face-to-face contact whenever possible.**

    Promotes understanding and independence.

4. **Provide for resident's privacy with curtain, screen, or door.**

    Maintains resident's right to privacy and dignity.

5. **Adjust bed to a safe working level, usually waist high. Lock bed wheels.**

    Prevents injury to you and to resident.

6. **Lower the head of bed. Move pillow to head of the bed.**

    When bed is flat, resident can be moved without working against gravity. Pillow prevents injury should resident hit the head of bed.

7. **Lower the side rail (if not already lowered) on side nearest you.**

8. **Stand by bed with feet apart. Face the resident.**

9. **Place one arm under resident's shoulder blades. Place other arm under resident's thighs. Use good body mechanics.**

    Putting your arm under resident's neck could cause injury.

10. **Ask resident to bend knees, brace feet on mattress, and push feet on the count of three.**

    Enables resident to help as much as possible and reduces strain on you.

11. **On three, shift body weight. Move resident while resident pushes with her feet (Fig. 5-44).**

    Communicating helps resident help you.

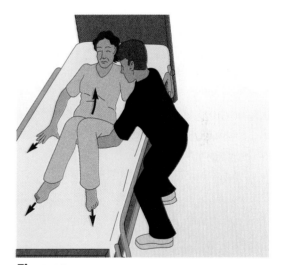

Fig. 5-44.

12. **Place pillow under resident's head.**

    Provides for resident's comfort.

13. **Return bed to appropriate position. Remove privacy measures.**

    Lowering the bed provides for resident's safety.

14. **Before leaving, place call light within resident's reach.**

    Allows resident to communicate with staff as necessary.

15. **Wash hands.**

    Provides for infection control.

5

Personal Care Skills

16. **Report any changes in resident to the nurse.**

    Provides nurse with information to assess resident.

17. **Document procedure using facility guidelines.**

    What you write is a legal record of what you did. If you don't document it, legally it didn't happen.

Moving a resident to the side of the bed

1. **Wash hands.**

    Provides for infection control.

2. **Identify yourself by name. Identify the resident by name.**

    Resident has right to know identity of his or her caregiver. Addressing resident by name shows respect and establishes correct identification.

3. **Explain procedure to resident. Speak clearly, slowly, and directly. Maintain face-to-face contact whenever possible.**

    Promotes understanding and independence.

4. **Provide for resident's privacy with curtain, screen, or door.**

    Maintains resident's right to privacy and dignity.

5. **Adjust the bed to a safe working level, usually waist high. Lock bed wheels (Fig. 5-45).**

    Prevents injury to you and to resident.

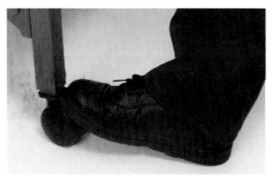

Fig. 5-45. Always lock the bed wheels before repositioning a resident in bed or transferring a resident to or from a bed.

6. **Lower the head of bed.**

    When bed is flat, resident can be moved without working against gravity.

7. **Gently slide your hands under the head and shoulders and move toward you**

(Fig. 5-46). Gently slide your hands under midsection and move toward you. Gently slide your hands under hips and legs and move toward you (Fig. 5-47).

Protects resident's skin.

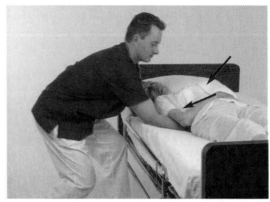

Fig. 5-46.

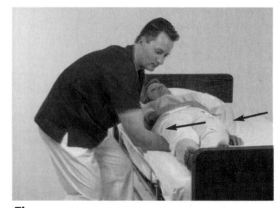

Fig. 5-47.

8. **Return bed to appropriate level. Remove privacy measures.**

    Lowering the bed provides for resident's safety.

9. **Before leaving, place call light within resident's reach.**

    Allows resident to communicate with staff as necessary.

10. **Wash hands.**

    Provides for infection control.

11. **Report any changes in resident to the nurse.**

    Provides nurse with information to assess resident.

12. **Document procedure using facility guidelines.**

    What you write is a legal record of what you did. If you don't document it, legally it didn't happen.

Turning a resident

1. **Wash hands.**
    Provides for infection control.

2. **Identify yourself by name. Identify the resident by name.**
    Resident has right to know identity of his or her caregiver. Addressing resident by name shows respect and establishes correct identification.

3. **Explain procedure to resident. Speak clearly, slowly, and directly. Maintain face-to-face contact whenever possible.**
    Promotes understanding and independence.

4. **Provide for resident's privacy with curtain, screen, or door.**
    Maintains resident's right to privacy and dignity.

5. **Adjust bed to a safe working level, usually waist high. Lock bed wheels.**
    Prevents injury to you and to resident.

6. **Lower the head of bed.**
    When bed is flat, resident can be moved without working against gravity.

7. **Stand on side of bed opposite to where person will be turned. The far side rail should be raised.**

8. **Lower side rail nearest you if it is up.**

9. **Move resident to side of bed nearest you using previous procedure.**
    Positions resident for turn.

    Turning resident away from you:

10. **Cross resident's arm over his or her chest. Move arm on side resident is being turned to out of the way. Cross leg nearest you over the far leg (Fig. 5-48).**

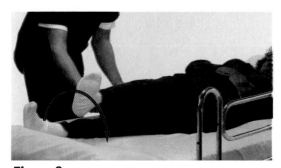

Fig. 5-48.

a. **Stand with feet about 12 inches apart. Bend your knees.**
Reduces your risk of injury. Promotes good body mechanics.

b. **Place one hand on the resident's shoulder. Place the other hand on the resident's nearest hip.**

c. **Gently push resident toward other side of bed. Shift your weight from your back leg to your front leg (Fig. 5-49).**

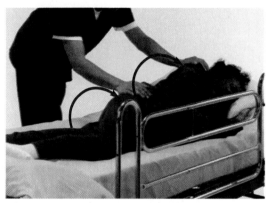

Fig. 5-49.

Turning resident toward you:

10. **Cross resident's arm over his or her chest. Move arm on side resident is being turned to out of the way. Cross leg furthest from you over the near leg.**

    a. **Stand with feet about 12 inches apart. Bend your knees.**
    Reduces your risk of injury. Promotes good body mechanics.

    b. **Place one hand on the resident's far shoulder. Place the other hand on the resident's far hip.**

    c. **Gently roll the resident toward you (Fig. 5-50). Your body will block resident and prevent her from rolling out of bed.**

11. **Position resident properly:**

*   **head supported by pillow**

*   **shoulder adjusted so resident is not lying on arm**

*   **top arm supported by pillow**

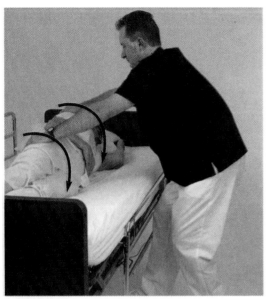

Fig. 5-50.

- back supported by supportive device
- top knee flexed
- supportive device between legs with top knee flexed; knee and ankle supported

12. **Return bed to appropriate level. Remove privacy measures.**
    Lowering the bed provides for resident's safety.

13. **Before leaving, place call light within resident's reach.**
    Allows resident to communicate with staff as necessary.

14. **Wash hands.**
    Provides for infection control.

15. **Report any changes in resident to the nurse.**
    Provides nurse with information to assess resident.

16. **Document procedure using facility guidelines.**
    What you write is a legal record of what you did. If you don't document it, legally it didn't happen.

Logrolling means moving a resident as a unit, without disturbing the alignment of the body. The head, back and legs must be kept in a straight line. This is necessary in cases of neck or back problems, spinal cord injuries, or back or hip surgeries. A draw sheet assists with moving. A draw sheet is an extra sheet placed on top of the bottom sheet when the bed is made.

Logrolling a resident with one assistant

Equipment: draw sheet, co-worker

1. **Wash hands.**
   Provides for infection control.

2. **Identify yourself by name. Identify the resident by name.**
   Resident has right to know identity of his or her caregiver. Addressing resident by name shows respect and establishes correct identification.

3. **Explain procedure to resident. Speak clearly, slowly, and directly. Maintain face-to-face contact whenever possible.**
   Promotes understanding and independence.

4. **Provide for resident's privacy with curtain, screen, or door.**
   Maintains resident's right to privacy and dignity.

5. **Adjust bed to a safe working level, usually waist high. Lock bed wheels.**
   Prevents injury to you and to resident.

6. **Lower the head of bed.**
   When bed is flat, resident can be moved without working against gravity.

7. **Lower the side rail on side closest to you.**

8. **Both co-workers stand on the same side of the bed. One person stands at the resident's head and shoulders. The other stands near the resident's midsection.**

9. **Place the resident's arms across his or her chest. Place a pillow between the knees.**

10. **Stand with feet about 12 inches apart. Bend your knees.**
    Reduces your risk of injury. Promotes good body mechanics.

11. **Grasp the draw sheet on the far side (Fig. 5-51).**

5

Personal Care Skills

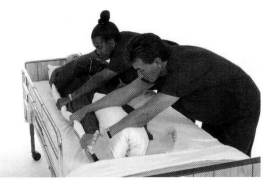

Fig. 5-51.

12. **On the count of three, gently roll the resident toward you. Turn the resident as a unit (Fig. 5-52).**
Work together for your safety and the resident's.

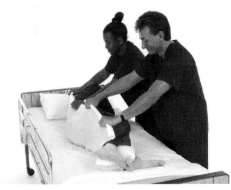

Fig. 5-52.

13. **Reposition resident comfortably.**
Maintains alignment.

14. **Return bed to appropriate level. Remove privacy measures.**
Lowering the bed provides for resident's safety.

15. **Before leaving, place call light within resident's reach.**
Allows resident to communicate with staff as necessary.

16. **Wash hands.**
Provides for infection control.

17. **Report any changes in resident to the nurse.**
Provides nurse with information to assess resident.

18. **Document procedure using facility guidelines.**
What you write is a legal record of what you did. If you don't document it, legally it didn't happen.

Before a resident who has been lying down stands up, she should dangle. To **dangle** means to sit up with the feet over the side of the bed to regain balance.

Assisting resident to sit up on side of bed: dangling

1. **Wash hands.**
Provides for infection control.

2. **Identify yourself by name. Identify the resident by name.**
Resident has right to know identity of his or her caregiver. Addressing resident by name shows respect and establishes correct identification.

3. **Explain procedure to resident. Speak clearly, slowly, and directly. Maintain face-to-face contact whenever possible.**
Promotes understanding and independence.

4. **Provide for resident's privacy with curtain, screen, or door.**
Maintains resident's right to privacy and dignity.

5. **Adjust bed height to lowest position. Lock bed wheels.**
Allows resident's feet to touch floor when sitting. Reduces chance of injury if resident falls.

6. **Raise the head of bed to sitting position.**
Resident can move without working against gravity.

7. **Place one arm under resident's shoulder blades. Place the other arm under resident's thighs (Fig. 5-53).**
Placing your arm under the resident's neck may cause injury.

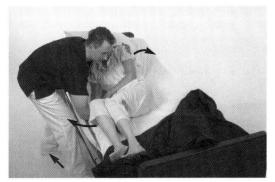

Fig. 5-53.

Personal Care Skills

5

8. **On the count of three, slowly turn resident into sitting position with legs dangling over side of bed (Fig. 5-54).**
Communicating helps resident help you.

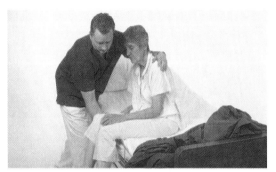

Fig. 5-54.

9. **Ask resident to hold onto edge of mattress with both hands. Assist resident to put on non-skid shoes or slippers.**
Prevents sliding on floor and protects resident's feet from contamination.

10. **Have resident dangle as long as ordered. Stay with the resident at all times. Check for dizziness. If resident feels dizzy or faint, help her lie down again. Tell the nurse at once.**
Change of position may cause dizziness due to a drop in blood pressure.

11. **Take vital signs as ordered (chapter 6).**

12. **Remove slippers or shoes.**

13. **Gently assist resident back into bed. Place one arm around resident's shoulders. Place the other arm under resident's knees. Slowly swing resident's legs onto bed.**

14. **Make sure resident is comfortable. Remove privacy measures.**

15. **Before leaving, place call light within resident's reach.**
Allows resident to communicate with staff as necessary.

16. **Wash hands.**
Provides for infection control.

17. **Report any changes in resident to the nurse.**
Provides nurse with information to assess resident.

18. **Document procedure using facility guidelines.**
What you write is a legal record of what you did. If you don't document it, legally it didn't happen.

Transfers allow a resident to move from one place to another. An example of a transfer is from the bed to the chair or toilet. One of the most important considerations during resident transfers is safety. In 2002, OSHA announced new ergonomic guidelines for transfers. **Ergonomics** is the practice of designing equipment and work tasks to suit the worker's abilities. OSHA now recommends that manual lifting of residents should be reduced in all cases and eliminated when possible. Manual lifting, transferring, and repositioning of residents may increase risks of pain and injury. For facilities, this means buying equipment to help aides perform these tasks. For NAs, this means using equipment properly. Always get help when you need it.

Some transfers require use of devices. A **transfer belt** is a safety device used to transfer residents who are weak, unsteady, or uncoordinated. It is called a "gait belt" when it is used to help residents walk. The belt is made of canvas or other heavy material. It sometimes has handles. It fits around the resident's waist outside his or her clothing. When putting a transfer belt on, leave room to insert four fingers under the belt. The belt gives you something firm to hold on to. Transfer belts cannot be used if a resident has fragile bones or recent fractures.

A sliding or transfer board may be used to help transfer residents who are unable to bear weight on their legs. Slide boards can be used for almost any transfer that involves moving from one sitting position to another. This includes transfers from a bed to a chair (Fig. 5-55).

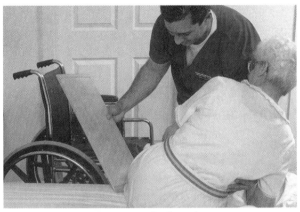

Fig. 5-55. A sliding or transfer board.

Wheelchairs/Geriatric Chairs

- Learn how a wheelchair works. You should know how to apply and release the brake and how to work the armrests and footrests. The wheelchair should be locked before helping a resident into or out of it (Fig. 5-56). After a transfer, a wheelchair should be unlocked.

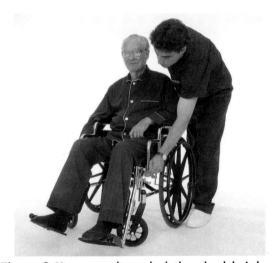

Fig. 5-56. You must always lock the wheelchair before a resident gets into or out of it.

- To open a standard wheelchair, pull on both sides. Make the armrests separate and the seat flatten. To close the wheelchair, lift the center of the seat. Pull upward until the chair collapses.

- When handling armrests and footrests, be very careful to prevent injury or skin tears. To remove an armrest, press a button, usually by the armrest, and lift it. To at-

tach an armrest, line up the buttons. Slip into place until the buttons click. To remove the footrest, locate the lever. Pull back, and pull the footrest off the knobs (Fig. 5-57). To re-attach the footrest, line up the knobs. Slide footrest into place until it clicks.

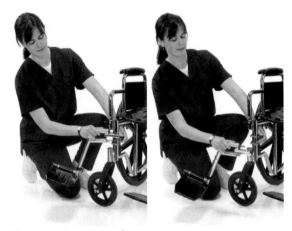

Fig. 5-57. Removing footrests.

- To lift or lower footrest, support the leg or foot. Squeeze lever and pull up or push down.

- Make sure the resident is safe and comfortable during transfers. When moving down a ramp, go backwards. The resident should face the top of the ramp, also going backwards. When using an elevator, turn the chair around before entering it, so the resident faces forward in the elevator.

- If the resident needs to be moved back in the wheelchair or geriatric chair (gerichair), go to the back of the chair. Gently reach forward and down under the resident's arms. Ask the resident to place his feet on the ground and push up. Gently pull the resident up in the chair while the resident pushes. Or, use another staff member to assist with the move.

- The tray table on geri-chairs can be heavy. Use caution when raising and lowering this table. Do not catch your fingers or the resident's fingers in the tray when attach-

5

ing or releasing the tray table. A locked tray on a geri-chair is considered a restraint. You must have a doctor's order to use it. It must be released every two hours for repositioning resident.

- Ask the resident how you can assist with wheelchairs. Some residents may only want you to bring the chair to the bedside. Others may need you to be more involved.

Falls

When a resident falls:

- Widen your stance and bring the resident's body close to you to break the fall. Bend your knees and support the resident as you lower her to the floor (Fig. 5-58).

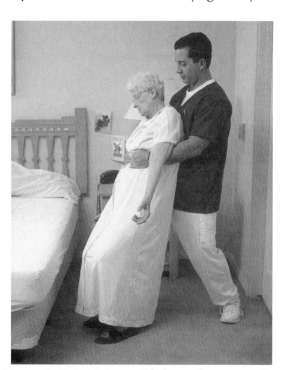

Fig. 5-58. Maintaining a wide base of support will help you assist a falling resident.

- Do not try to reverse or stop a fall. You or the resident can suffer worse injuries if you try to stop it rather than break it.

- Call for help. Do not attempt to get the resident up after the fall. Follow facility policy. Take resident's vital signs. Report the fall to nurse so that the incident report can be prepared.

Transferring a resident from bed to wheelchair

Equipment: wheelchair, transfer belt, non-skid footwear

1. **Wash hands.**
   Provides for infection control.

2. **Identify yourself by name. Identify the resident by name.**
   Resident has right to know identity of his or her caregiver. Addressing resident by name shows respect and establishes correct identification.

3. **Explain procedure to resident. Speak clearly, slowly, and directly. Maintain face-to-face contact whenever possible.**
   Promotes understanding and independence.

4. **Provide for resident's privacy with curtain, screen, or door.**
   Maintains resident's right to privacy and dignity.

5. **Remove wheelchair footrests close to the bed.**

6. **Place wheelchair near the head of the bed with arm of the wheelchair almost touching the bed. Wheelchair should be placed on resident's stronger, or unaffected, side.**
   Unaffected side supports weight.

7. **Lock wheelchair wheels.**
   Wheel locks prevent chair from moving.

8. **Raise the head of the bed. Adjust bed level. The height of the bed should be equal to or slightly higher than the chair. Lock bed wheels.**
   Prevents injury to you and to resident.

9. **Assist resident to sitting position with feet flat on the floor.**

10. **Put non-skid footwear on resident and securely fasten.**
    Promotes resident's safety. Reduces risk of falls.

11. *With transfer (gait) belt:*
    a. Stand in front of resident.
    b. Stand with feet about 12 inches apart. Bend your knees.
    Reduces risk of injury. Promotes good body mechanics.

c. Place belt around resident's waist. Grasp belt securely on both sides.

Without transfer belt:

a. Stand in front of resident.

b. Stand with feet about 12 inches apart. Bend your knees.

Reduces your risk of injury. Promotes good body mechanics.

c. Place your arms around resident's torso under the arms. Ask resident to place her hands on your shoulders if possible, or use bed to push up with.

12. Provide instructions to allow resident to help with transfer. Instructions may include:

"When you start to stand, push with your hands against the bed."

"Once standing, if you're able, you can take small steps in the direction of the chair."

"Once standing, reach for the chair with your stronger hand."

13. With your legs, brace resident's lower legs to prevent slipping (Fig. 5-59).

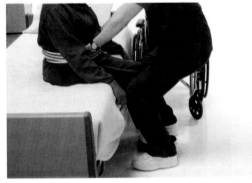

Fig. 5-59.

14. Count to three to alert resident.

15. On three, slowly help resident to stand.

Communicating helps resident help you.

16. Help resident to pivot to front of wheelchair with back of resident's legs against wheelchair (Fig. 5-60).

Pivoting is safer than twisting.

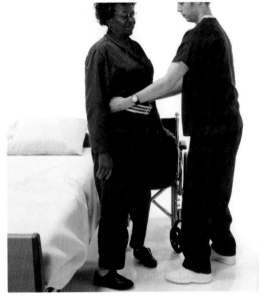

Fig. 5-60.

17. Ask resident to put hands on wheelchair arm rests if able.

18. Gently lower resident into wheelchair.

19. Reposition resident with hips touching back of wheelchair. Remove transfer belt, if used.

Using full seat of chair is safest position.

20. Attach footrests. Place resident's feet on footrests.

Protects feet and ankles.

21. Remove privacy measures.

22. Before leaving, place call light within resident's reach.

Allows resident to communicate with staff as necessary.

23. Wash hands.

Provides for infection control.

24. Report any changes in resident to the nurse.

Provides nurse with information to assess resident.

25. Document procedure using facility guidelines.

What you write is a legal record of what you did. If you don't document it, legally it didn't happen.

👁 *You must lock the wheels on both the wheelchair and the bed before transferring.*

Mechanical Lifts

You may help the resident with many types of transfers using the mechanical or hydraulic lift if you are trained to do so. This lift avoids wear and tear on your body. Lifts help prevent injury to you and the resident.

• Never use equipment you have not been trained to use. You or your resident could get hurt if you use lifting equipment improperly.

• There are many different types of mechanical lifts (Fig. 5-61). The names of these lifts vary. "Hydraulic," "power," "standing," "heavy duty," "pool and bath," etc. are some of the names you may hear. You must be trained on the specific lift you will be using. Using these devices helps prevent common workplace injuries. Follow the care plan. Use provided equipment correctly, according to facility policy. Some facilities may require two caregivers to assist when using a specific lift.

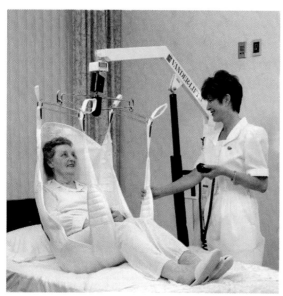

Fig. 5-61. This is one type of mechanical lift. (Photo courtesy of VANCARE Inc., 800-694-4525.)

Some facilities require two staff members for all transfers using mechanical lifts. Follow facility policy.

Transferring a resident using a mechanical lift

This is a basic procedure for transferring a resident using a mechanical lift with the type of sling shown in the photo. Other lifts may have different procedures.

Equipment: wheelchair or chair, co-worker, mechanical or hydraulic lift

1. **Wash hands.**
   Provides for infection control.

2. **Identify yourself by name. Identify the resident by name.**
   Resident has right to know identity of his or her caregiver. Addressing resident by name shows respect and establishes correct identification.

3. **Explain procedure to resident. Speak clearly, slowly, and directly. Maintain face-to-face contact whenever possible.**
   Promotes understanding and independence.

4. **Provide for resident's privacy with curtain, screen, or door.**
   Maintains resident's right to privacy and dignity.

5. **Lock bed wheels.**
   Wheel locks prevent bed from moving.

6. **Position wheelchair next to bed. Lock brakes.**
   Wheel locks prevent chair from moving.

7. **Help the resident turn to one side of the bed. Position the sling under the resident, with the edge next to the resident's back. Fanfold if necessary. Fanfolding means folding several times into pleats. Make the bottom of the sling even with the resident's knees (some slings only come to the top of the buttocks). Help the resident roll back to the middle of the bed. Spread out the fanfolded edge of the sling.**

8. **Roll the mechanical lift to bedside. Make sure the base is opened to its widest point. Push the base of the lift under the bed.**

9. Place the overhead bar directly over the resident.

10. With the resident lying on her back, attach one set of straps to each side of the sling. Attach one set of straps to the overhead bar. If available, have a co-worker support the resident at the head, shoulders, and knees while being lifted. The resident's arms should be folded across her chest. If the device has "S" hooks, they should face away from resident. Make sure all straps are connected properly.

11. Following manufacturer's instructions, raise the resident two inches above the bed. Pause a moment for the resident to gain balance.

12. If available, a lifting partner can help support and guide the resident's body. You can then move the lift so that the resident is positioned over the chair or wheelchair.
Having another person help promotes safety during the transfer and lessens chance of injury.

13. Slowly lower the resident into the chair or wheelchair. Push down gently on the resident's knees to help the resident into a sitting position.

14. Undo the straps from the overhead bar. Leave the sling in place for transfer back to bed (some slings can be easily removed when resident is seated).

15. Be sure the resident is seated comfortably and correctly in the chair or wheelchair. Remove privacy measures.

16. Before leaving, place call light within resident's reach.
Allows resident to communicate with staff as necessary.

17. Wash your hands.
Provides for infection control.

18. Report any changes in resident to the nurse.
Provides nurse with information to assess resident.

19. Document procedure using facility guidelines.
What you write is a legal record of what you did. If you don't document it, legally it didn't happen.

six

Basic Nursing Skills

Unit 1. Explain admission, transfer, and discharge of a resident

When a resident is admitted to a nursing home, the nursing assistant has an important role. This includes supporting residents emotionally. Moving into a nursing home is a big change. A resident may feel fear, loss, anger, and uncertainty (Fig. 6-1). Because change is difficult, staff must communicate with new residents. Explain what to expect during the process. Answer any questions a resident has. Ask questions to find out a resident's personal preferences and routines.

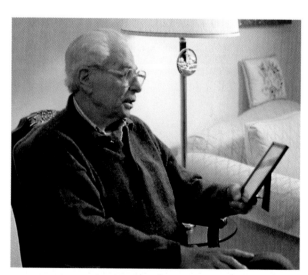

Fig. 6-1. **A new resident may have just lost someone very close to him. Be supportive. Listen to him if he wants to talk.**

Admission is often the first time you meet a new resident. This is a time of first impressions. Make sure a resident has a good impression of you and your facility. Your facility will have a procedure for admitting residents to their new home. These guidelines will help make the experience as pleasant and successful as possible.

Guidelines
Admission

- Prepare the room before the resident arrives so he or she will feel expected and welcome. Know the condition of the resident. Know if he or she is bed-bound or is able to walk.

- Introduce yourself. Explain your position. Always call the person by his formal name until he tells you what he wants to be called.

- Never rush the process or the new resident. He should not feel like he is an inconvenience.

- Make every effort to see that the new resident feels welcome, comfortable, and wanted.

- Explain day-to-day life in the facility. Offer to take the resident on a tour (Fig. 6-2).

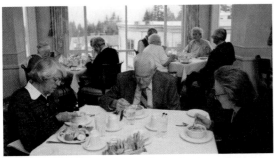

Fig. 6-2. Make sure you include the location of the dining room when taking a new resident on a tour.

- Introduce the resident to other residents and staff members you see (Fig. 6-3). Introduce the roommate if there is one.

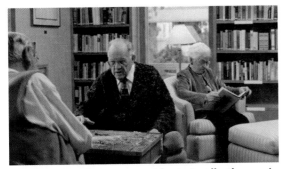

Fig. 6-3. Introduce new residents to all other residents you see.

- Handle personal items carefully and respectfully. These items are special things he has chosen to bring with him. When setting up the room, ask him what he likes. Place personal items where the resident wants them (Fig. 6-4).

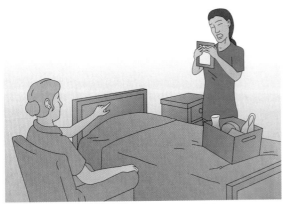

Fig. 6-4. Handle a resident's personal items carefully. Set up the room according to her preference.

- Follow your facility's rules regarding your tasks.

RA *Upon admission, residents must be informed of their rights and be provided with a written copy of these rights. This includes rights about personal funds and the right to file a complaint with the state survey agency.*

Admitting a resident

Equipment: may include admission paperwork (checklist and inventory form), gloves and vital signs equipment

Often an admission kit will contain a urine specimen cup and transport bag, and personal care items, such as bath basin, water pitcher, drinking glass, toothpaste and soap.

1. **Wash hands.**
   Provides for infection control.

2. **Identify yourself by name. Identify the resident by name.**
   Resident has right to know identity of his or her caregiver. Addressing resident by name shows respect and establishes correct identification.

3. **Explain procedure to resident. Speak clearly, slowly, and directly. Maintain face-to-face contact whenever possible.**
   Promotes understanding and independence.

4. **Provide for resident's privacy with curtain, screen, or door. If the family is present, ask them to step outside until the admission process is over.**
   Maintains resident's right to privacy and dignity.

5. **If part of facility procedure, do these things:**

   Take the resident's height and weight (see unit 3).

   Take the resident's baseline vital signs (unit 2). Baseline signs are initial values that can then be compared to future measurements.

   Obtain a urine specimen if required (unit 5).

   Complete the paperwork. Take an inventory of all the personal items.

6

Basic Nursing Skills

Help the resident to put personal items away. Label personal items according to facility policy.

Provide fresh water.

6. **Show the resident to the room and bathroom. Explain how to work the bed (and television if there is one). Show the resident how to work the call light and explain its use.**
   Promotes resident's safety.

7. **Introduce the resident to his roommate, if there is one. Introduce other residents and staff.**
   Makes resident feel more comfortable.

8. **Make sure resident is comfortable. Remove privacy measures.**

9. **Before leaving, place call light within resident's reach.**
   Allows resident to communicate with staff as necessary.

10. **Wash hands.**
    Provides for infection control.

11. **Document procedure using facility guidelines.**
    What you write is a legal record of what you did. If you don't document it, legally it didn't happen.

Residents may be transferred to a different area of the facility. In cases of acute illness, they may be transferred to a hospital. Change is difficult. This is especially true when a person has an illness or his condition gets worse. Make the transfer as smooth as possible for the resident. Try to lessen the stress. Inform him of the transfer as soon as possible. He can then begin to adjust to the idea. Explain how, where, when and why the transfer will occur.

For example, "Mr. Jones, you will be moving to a private room. You will be transferred to your new room in a wheelchair. This will happen on Wednesday around 10 a.m. The staff will take good care of you and your things. We will make sure you are comfortable. Do you have any questions?"

Residents often worry about losing their belongings. Involve them with the packing process if appropriate. For example, let them see the empty closet, drawers, etc.

RЯ *Residents have the right to receive notice of any room or roommate change.*

Transferring a resident

Equipment: may include a wheelchair, cart for belongings, the medical record, all of the resident's personal care items

1. **Wash hands.**
   Provides for infection control.

2. **Identify yourself by name. Identify the resident by name.**
   Resident has right to know identity of his or her caregiver. Addressing resident by name shows respect and establishes correct identification.

3. **Explain procedure to resident. Speak clearly, slowly, and directly. Maintain face-to-face contact whenever possible.**
   Promotes understanding and independence.

4. **Collect items to be moved onto the cart. Take them to the new location. If the resident is going into the hospital, they may be placed in temporary storage.**

5. **Help the resident into the wheelchair (stretcher may be used).**

6. **Transfer resident to his new unit or room.**

7. **Introduce new residents and staff.**
   Makes resident feel more comfortable.

8. **Assist the resident to put personal items away.**

9. **Make sure the resident is comfortable.**

10. **Before leaving, place call light within resident's reach.**
    Allows resident to communicate with staff as necessary.

11. **Wash hands.**
    Provides for infection control.

12. **Report any changes in resident to the nurse.**
    Provides nurse with information to assess resident.

13. **Document procedure using facility guidelines.**
    What you write is a legal record of what you did. If you don't document it, legally it didn't happen.

The day of discharge is usually a happy day for a resident who is going home. You will collect the resident's belongings and pack them. Know the resident's condition. Find out if he will be using a wheelchair or stretcher for discharge. Ask the resident which personal care items to include. Be positive. Assure the resident he is ready for this important change. He may have doubts about not being cared for at the facility anymore. Remind him that his doctor believes he is ready.

The nurse may cover important information with the resident and family. Some of these areas may be discussed:

- future doctor or physical therapy appointments (Fig. 6-5)

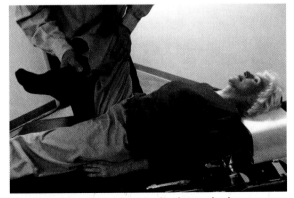

Fig. 6-5. After a resident is discharged, she may continue to receive physical therapy.

- medications
- the ambulation instructions from the doctor

- any restrictions on activities
- special exercises to keep the resident functioning at the highest level
- any special dietary requirements
- community resources

Discharging a resident

Equipment: may include a wheelchair, cart for belongings, the discharge paperwork, including the inventory list done on admission, all of the resident's personal care items

1. **Wash hands.**
   Provides for infection control.

2. **Identify yourself by name. Identify the resident by name.**
   Resident has right to know identity of his or her caregiver. Addressing resident by name shows respect and establishes correct identification.

3. **Explain procedure to resident. Speak clearly, slowly, and directly. Maintain face-to-face contact whenever possible.**
   Promotes understanding and independence.

4. **Provide for resident's privacy with curtain, screen, or door.**
   Maintains resident's right to privacy and dignity.

5. **Compare the checklist to the items there. If all items are there, ask the resident to sign.**

6. **Put the items to be taken onto the cart and take them to pick-up area.**

7. **Help the resident dress and then help him into the wheelchair (stretcher may be used for some residents).**

8. **Help the resident to say his goodbyes to the staff and residents.**

9. **Take resident to the pick-up area. Help him into vehicle. You are responsible for the resident until he is safely in the car and the door is closed and the seat belt is on.**

10. **Wash hands.**
    Provides for infection control.

11. Document procedure using facility guidelines.

What you write is a legal record of what you did. If you don't document it, legally it didn't happen.

📋 *The survey team will make sure that each resident has his or her rights protected and needs met during admission and/or discharge. This is true whether a resident is a private pay resident or on public aid. Staff must provide proper care and services regardless of who pays the bills.*

Unit 2. Explain the importance of monitoring vital signs

You will monitor, document, and report your residents' vital signs. Vital signs are important. They show how well the vital organs of the body, such as the heart and lungs, are working. They consist of the following:

- taking the body temperature
- counting the pulse
- counting the rate of respirations
- taking the blood pressure
- observing and reporting level of pain

Watching for changes in vital signs is very important. Changes can indicate a resident's condition is worsening. Always notify the nurse if:

- the resident is running a fever
- the resident has a respiratory or pulse rate that is too rapid or too slow
- the resident's blood pressure changes
- the resident's pain is worse or is not relieved by pain management

📋 *The survey team will make sure that staff take vital signs as indicated in the plan of care so that the resident's well-being and functioning are at their highest levels.*

Normal Ranges for Adult Vital Signs

Temperature:	Fahrenheit	Celsius
Oral	97.6°-99.6°	36.5°-37.5°
Rectal	98.6°-100.6°	37.0°-38.1°
Axillary	96.6°-98.6°	36.0°-37.0°

Pulse: 60-90 beats per minute

Respirations: 12-20 respirations per minute

Blood Pressure:

Normal:

> Systolic 100-119
>
> Diastolic 60-79

Prehypertension:

> Systolic 120-139
>
> Diastolic 80-89

High:

> 140/90 or above *

** Millions of people whose blood pressure was considered normal (120/80) now fall into the "prehypertension" range. **Prehypertension** means that the person does not have high blood pressure now but is likely to have it in the future. This is based on the new, more aggressive high blood pressure guidelines from the Seventh Report of the Joint National Committee (JNC 7) on Prevention, Detection, Evaluation, and Treatment of High Blood Pressure (2003).*

Temperature

Body temperature is normally very close to 98.6° F (Fahrenheit) or 37° C (Celsius). Body temperature is a balance between the heat created by our bodies and the heat lost to the environment. Increases in body temperature may indicate an infection or disease. There are four sites for taking body temperature:

1. the mouth (oral)
2. the rectum (rectal)
3. the armpit (axillary)
4. the ear (tympanic)

The different sites require different thermometers. Temperatures are most often taken orally. Do not take an oral temperature on a person who:

- is unconscious
- is using oxygen
- is confused or disoriented
- is paralyzed from stroke
- has facial trauma
- is likely to have a seizure
- has a nasogastric tube (chapter 7)
- is younger than six years old
- has sores, redness, swelling, or pain in the mouth
- has an injury to the face or neck

Types of thermometers are

- Mercury-free (Fig. 6-6)

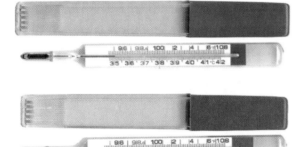

Fig. 6-6. A mercury-free oral thermometer and a mercury-free rectal thermometer. Thermometers are usually color-coded to tell you which is an oral and which is a rectal thermometer. Oral thermometers are usually green or blue. Rectal thermometers are usually red. (Photos courtesy of RG Medical Diagnostics of Southfield, MI.)

- Mercury glass *
- Battery-powered, digital (Fig. 6-7), or electronic (Fig. 6-8)

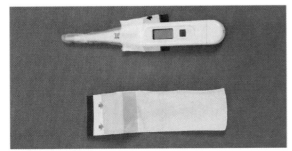

Fig. 6-7. A digital thermometer.

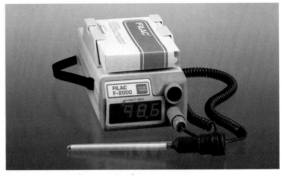

Fig. 6-8. An electronic thermometer.

- Tympanic (ear) (Fig. 6-9)

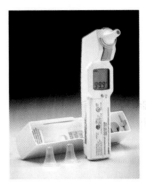

Fig. 6-9. A tympanic thermometer.

* Using glass bulb or mercury thermometers to take oral or rectal temperatures used to be common. Because mercury is dangerous, many facilities now discourage the use of mercury. Many states have passed laws to ban the sale of mercury thermometers. Mercury-free thermometers are considered much safer.

If using a mercury glass thermometer, handle it with care. If the thermometer breaks, report it to the nurse immediately. When cleaning a mercury glass thermometer, wipe it with tissues first. Use lukewarm or cool water to clean it. Never use hot water. Hot water can heat the mercury and break the thermometer.

Mercury-free thermometers are slightly larger than glass bulb thermometers. They operate identically. Numbers on the thermometer let you read the temperature after it registers. Most thermometers show the

6

Basic Nursing Skills

temperature in degrees Fahrenheit (F). Each long line represents one degree. Each short line represents two-tenths of a degree. Some thermometers show the temperature in degrees Celsius (C). The long lines represent one degree. The short lines represent one-tenth of a degree. The small arrow points to the normal temperature: 98.6° F and 37° C (Fig. 6-10).

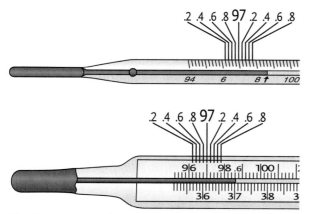

Fig. 6-10. You read a mercury glass and a mercury-free thermometer the same way.

There is a range of normal temperatures. Some people's temperatures normally run low. Others in good health will run slightly higher. Normal temperature readings also vary by the method used to take the temperature. A rectal temperature is generally considered to be the most accurate.

Taking and recording oral temperature

Do not take an oral temperature on a resident who has eaten or drunk fluids in the last 10–20 minutes.
Equipment: mercury-free, digital, or electronic thermometer, gloves, disposable plastic sheath/cover for thermometers, tissues, pen and paper

1. **Wash hands.**
    Provides for infection control.

2. **Identify yourself by name. Identify the resident by name.**
    Resident has right to know identity of his or her caregiver. Addressing resident by name shows respect and establishes correct identification.

3. **Explain procedure to resident. Speak clearly, slowly, and directly. Maintain face-to-face contact whenever possible.**
    Promotes understanding and independence.

4. **Provide for resident's privacy with curtain, screen, or door.**
    Maintains resident's right to privacy and dignity.

5. **Put on gloves.**

Using a mercury-free thermometer:

6. **Hold thermometer by stem.**
    Holding the stem end prevents contamination of the bulb end.

7. **Before inserting thermometer in resident's mouth, shake thermometer down to below the lowest number (at least below 96°F or 35°C). To shake thermometer down, hold it at the side opposite the bulb with the thumb and two fingers. With a snapping motion of the wrist, shake the thermometer (Fig. 6-11). Stand away from furniture and walls while doing so.**
    The thermometer reading must be below the resident's actual temperature.

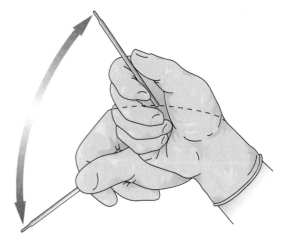

Fig. 6-11.

8. **Put on disposable sheath, if applicable. Insert bulb end of thermometer into resident's mouth. Place it under tongue and to one side (Fig. 6-12). Resident should breathe through his or her nose.**
    The thermometer measures heat from blood vessels under the tongue.

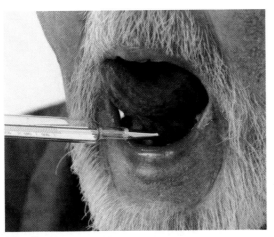

Fig. 6-12.

9. Tell resident to hold thermometer in mouth with lips closed. Assist as necessary. Ask the resident not to bite down or to talk.
   The lips hold the thermometer in position. If broken, injury to the mouth may occur.

10. Leave thermometer in place for at least three minutes.
    More time may be required if resident opens mouth to breathe or talk.

11. Remove the thermometer. Wipe with tissue from stem to bulb or remove sheath. Dispose of tissue or sheath.
    Reduces contamination.

12. Hold thermometer at eye level. Rotate until line appears. Roll thermometer between your thumb and forefinger. Read temperature. Remember temperature.

13. Rinse the thermometer in lukewarm water. Dry. Return it to plastic case or container.

Using a digital thermometer:

6. Put on disposable sheath.

7. Turn on thermometer. Wait until "ready" sign appears.

8. Insert end of digital thermometer into resident's mouth. Place under tongue and to one side.

9. Leave in place until thermometer blinks or beeps.

10. Remove the thermometer.

11. Read temperature on display screen. Remember temperature.

12. Using a tissue, remove and dispose of sheath.
    Reduces risk of contamination.

13. Replace thermometer in case.

Using an electronic thermometer:

6. Remove probe from base unit.

7. Put on probe cover.

8. Insert end of electronic thermometer into resident's mouth. Place under tongue and to one side.

9. Leave in place until you hear a tone or see a flashing or steady light.

10. Read the temperature on the display screen.

11. Remove the probe. Press the eject button to discard the cover (Fig. 6-13).

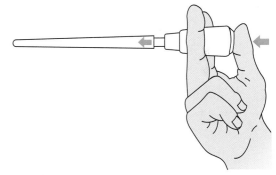

Fig. 6-13.

12. Remember temperature.

13. Return the probe to the holder.

Final steps:

14. Remove and dispose of gloves.

15. Immediately record resident's name, temperature, date, time, and method used (oral).
    Record temperature immediately so you won't forget. Care plans are made based on your report.

16. Wash hands.
    Provides for infection control.

6

Basic Nursing Skills

17. **Before leaving, place call light within resident's reach.**

    Allows resident to communicate with staff as necessary.

18. **Report any changes in resident to the nurse.**

    Provides nurse with information to assess resident.

19. **Document procedure using facility guidelines.**

    What you write is a legal record of what you did. If you don't document it, legally it didn't happen.

You need the resident's cooperation to take a rectal temperature. Always explain what you will do before beginning. Ask the resident to hold still. Reassure him that the task will only take a few minutes. **Hold onto the thermometer at all times.**

Taking and recording rectal temperature

Equipment: rectal mercury-free or digital thermometer, lubricant, gloves, tissue, disposable plastic sheath/ cover, pen and paper

1. **Wash hands.**

    Provides for infection control.

2. **Identify yourself by name. Identify resident by name.**

    Resident has right to know identity of his or her caregiver. Addressing resident by name shows respect and establishes correct identification.

3. **Explain procedure to resident. Speak clearly, slowly, and directly. Maintain face-to-face contact whenever possible.**

    Promotes understanding and independence.

4. **Provide for resident's privacy with curtain, screen, or door.**

    Maintains resident's right to privacy and dignity.

5. **If the bed is adjustable, adjust to a safe level, usually waist high. If the bed is movable, lock bed wheels.**

    Promotes safety.

6. **Help the resident to left-lying (Sims') position (Fig. 6-14).**

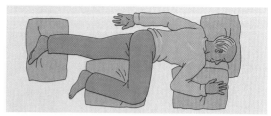

Fig. 6-14.

7. **Fold back linens to expose only the rectal area.**

8. **Put on gloves.**

9. *Mercury-free thermometer:* **Hold thermometer by stem.**

    Digital thermometer: **Apply probe cover.**

10. *Mercury-free thermometer:* **Shake thermometer down to below the lowest number.**

11. **Apply small amount of lubricant to tip of bulb or probe cover (or apply pre-lubricated cover).**

12. **Separate the buttocks. Gently insert thermometer one inch into rectum (Fig. 6-15). Stop if you meet resistance. Do not force the thermometer in the rectum.**

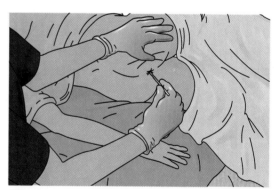

Fig. 6-15.

13. **Replace sheet over buttocks. Hold onto the thermometer at all times.**

14. *Mercury-free thermometer:* **Hold thermometer in place for at least three minutes.**

    Digital thermometer: **Hold thermometer in place until thermometer blinks or beeps.**

15. Gently remove the thermometer. Wipe with tissue from stem to bulb or remove sheath. Dispose of tissue or sheath.

16. Read thermometer at eye level as you would for an oral temperature. Remember temperature.

17. *Mercury-free thermometer:* Rinse thermometer in lukewarm water. Dry it. Return it to plastic case or container. If using a mercury/glass thermometer, store it away from a heat source.

    Digital thermometer: Throw away probe cover. Return thermometer to storage area.
    Reduces risk of contamination.

18. Remove and dispose of gloves.

19. Immediately record resident's name, temperature, date, time, and method used (rectal).
    Record temperature immediately so you won't forget. Care plans are made based on your report.

20. Wash hands.
    Provides for infection control.

21. Make resident comfortable.

22. Before leaving, place call light within resident's reach.
    Allows resident to communicate with staff as necessary.

23. Report any changes in resident to the nurse.
    Provides nurse with information to assess resident.

24. Document procedure using facility guidelines.
    What you write is a legal record of what you did. If you don't document it, legally it didn't happen.

Tympanic thermometers can take fast and accurate temperature readings. The short tip of the thermometer will only go into the ear one-quarter to one-half inch. Follow the manufacturer's instructions.

Taking and recording tympanic temperature

Equipment: tympanic thermometer, gloves, disposable probe sheath/cover, pen and paper

1. Wash hands.
   Provides for infection control.

2. Identify yourself by name. Identify the resident by name.
   Resident has right to know identity of his or her caregiver. Addressing resident by name shows respect and establishes correct identification.

3. Explain procedure to resident. Speak clearly, slowly, and directly. Maintain face-to-face contact whenever possible.
   Promotes understanding and independence.

4. Provide for resident's privacy with curtain, screen, or door.
   Maintains resident's right to privacy and dignity.

5. Put on gloves.

6. Put a disposable sheath over earpiece of the thermometer.
   Protects equipment. Reduces risk of contamination.

7. Position the resident's head so that the ear is in front of you. Straighten the ear canal by pulling up and back on the outside edge of the ear (Fig. 6-16). Insert the covered probe into the ear canal. Press the button.

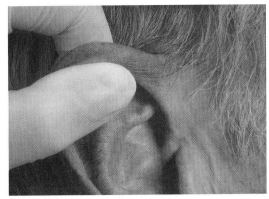

Fig. 6-16.

8. Hold thermometer in place until thermometer blinks or beeps.

9. Read temperature. Remember temperature.

10. Dispose of sheath. Return thermometer to storage or to the battery charger if thermometer is rechargeable.

11. Remove and dispose of gloves.

12. Immediately record resident's name, temperature, date, time, and method used (tympanic).

    Record temperature immediately so you won't forget. Care plans are made based on your report.

13. Wash hands.

    Provides for infection control.

14. Make resident comfortable.

15. Before leaving, place call light within resident's reach.

    Allows resident to communicate with staff as necessary.

16. Report any changes in resident to the nurse.

    Provides nurse with information to assess resident.

17. Document procedure using facility guidelines.

    What you write is a legal record of what you did. If you don't document it, legally it didn't happen.

Axillary temperatures are much less reliable than temperatures taken at other sites. The axillary site is usually used as a last resort.

Taking and recording axillary temperature

Equipment: mercury-free, digital, or electronic thermometer, gloves, tissues, disposable sheath/cover, pen and paper

1. Wash hands.

    Provides for infection control.

2. Identify yourself by name. Identify resident by name.

    Resident has right to know identity of his or her caregiver. Addressing resident by name shows respect and establishes correct identification.

3. Explain procedure to resident. Speak clearly, slowly, and directly. Maintain face-to-face contact whenever possible.

    Promotes understanding and independence.

4. Provide for resident's privacy with curtain, screen, or door.

    Maintains resident's right to privacy and dignity.

5. If the bed is adjustable, adjust bed to safe level, usually waist high. If the bed is movable, lock bed wheels.

    Promotes safety and good body mechanics.

6. Put on gloves.

7. Remove resident's arm from sleeve of gown. Wipe axillary area with tissues.

    This removes moisture from axillary area.

Using a mercury-free thermometer:

8. Hold thermometer at stem end and shake down to below the lowest number.

9. Put on disposable sheath, if applicable.

10. Place bulb end of thermometer in center of armpit. Fold resident's arm over chest.

    Puts thermometer against blood vessels to get the reading.

11. Hold thermometer in place, with the arm close against the side, for 10 minutes (Fig. 6-17).

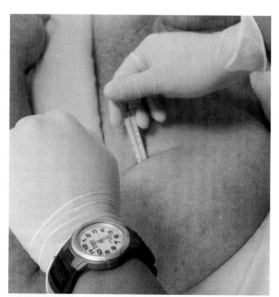

Fig. 6-17.

12. Remove the thermometer. Wipe with tissue from stem to bulb or remove sheath. Dispose of tissue or sheath.
Reduces risk of contamination.

13. Hold thermometer at eye level. Rotate until line appears. Read temperature. Remember temperature.

14. Clean thermometer and/or return it to container for used thermometers.

Using a digital thermometer:

8. Put on disposable sheath. Turn on thermometer. Wait until "ready" sign appears.

9. Position end of digital thermometer in center of armpit. Fold resident's arm over chest.
Puts thermometer against blood vessels to get the reading.

10. Hold in place until thermometer blinks or beeps.

11. Remove the thermometer.

12. Read temperature on display screen. Remember temperature.

13. Using a tissue, remove and dispose of sheath.
Reduces risk of contamination.

14. Replace thermometer in case.

Using an electronic thermometer:

8. Remove probe from base unit.

9. Put on probe cover.

10. Position end of electronic thermometer in center of armpit. Fold resident's arm over chest.
Puts thermometer against blood vessels to get the reading.

11. Leave in place until you hear a tone or see a flashing or steady light.

12. Read the temperature on the display screen. Remember temperature.

13. Remove the probe. Press the eject button to discard the cover.

14. Return the probe to the holder.

Final steps:

15. Put resident's arm back into sleeve of gown. Make resident comfortable.

16. Remove and dispose of gloves.

17. Immediately record resident's name, temperature, date, time, and method used (axillary).
Record temperature immediately so you won't forget. Care plans are made based on your report.

18. Wash hands.
Provides for infection control.

19. Return bed to proper position. Remove privacy measures.

20. Before leaving, place call light within resident's reach.
Allows resident to communicate with staff as necessary.

21. Report any changes in resident to the nurse.
Provides nurse with information to assess resident.

22. Document procedure according to facility guidelines.
What you write is a legal record of what you did. If you don't document it, legally it didn't happen.

Pulse

The pulse is the number of heartbeats per minute. The beat that you feel at certain pulse points in the body represents the wave of blood moving. This is a result of the heart pumping. The most common site for checking the pulse is on the inside of the wrist, where the radial artery runs just beneath the skin. This is called the **radial pulse**.

The **brachial pulse** is the pulse inside of the elbow. It is about 1–1½ inches above the elbow. The radial and brachial pulse are involved in taking blood pressure. Blood pressure is explained later in this chapter. Other common pulse sites are shown in Fig. 6-18.

6

Basic Nursing Skills

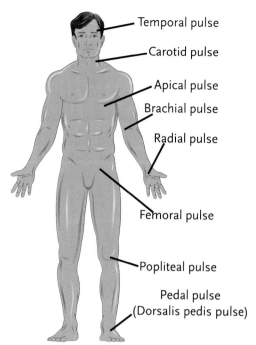

Temporal pulse
Carotid pulse
Apical pulse
Brachial pulse
Radial pulse
Femoral pulse
Popliteal pulse
Pedal pulse
(Dorsalis pedis pulse)

Fig. 6-18. Common pulse sites.

For adults, the normal pulse rate is 60–90 beats per minute. Small children have faster pulses, in the range of 100–120 beats per minute. A newborn baby's pulse may be as high as 120–140 beats per minute. Many things can affect the pulse rate. Some are exercise, fear, anger, anxiety, heat, medications, and pain. An unusually high or low rate may not indicate disease, but sometimes the pulse rate can be a signal of serious illness. A rapid pulse may result from fever, infection, or heart failure. A slow or weak pulse may indicate dehydration, infection, or shock.

Respirations

Respiration is the process of breathing air into the lungs, or **inspiration**, and exhaling air out of the lungs, or **expiration**. Each respiration consists of an inspiration and an expiration. The chest rises during inspiration and falls during expiration.

The normal respiration rate for adults ranges from 12–20 breaths per minute. Infants and children have a faster respiratory rate. Infants can breathe normally at a

rate of 30–40 respirations per minute. People may breathe more quickly if they know they are being observed. Because of this, count respirations immediately after taking the pulse. Keep your fingers on the resident's wrist or the stethoscope over the heart. Do not make it obvious that you are observing the resident's breathing.

Taking and recording radial pulse and counting and recording respirations

Equipment: watch with a second hand, pen and paper

1. **Wash hands.**
    Provides for infection control.

2. **Identify yourself by name. Identify the resident by name.**
    Resident has right to know identity of his or her caregiver. Addressing resident by name shows respect and establishes correct identification.

3. **Explain procedure to resident. Speak clearly, slowly, and directly. Maintain face-to-face contact whenever possible.**
    Promotes understanding and independence.

4. **Provide for resident's privacy with curtain, screen, or door.**
    Maintains resident's right to privacy and dignity.

5. **Place fingertips on thumb side of resident's wrist to locate pulse (Fig. 6-19).**

6. **Count beats for one full minute.**

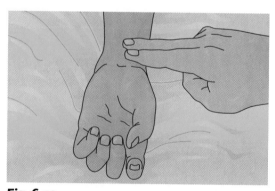

Fig. 6-19.

7. **Keep your fingertips on the resident's wrist. Count respirations for one full minute. Observe for the pattern and character of the resident's breathing.**

Normal breathing is smooth and quiet.
Count will be more accurate if resident does not know you are counting his respirations.

8. **Record pulse rate, date, time and method used (radial). Record the respiratory rate and the pattern or character of breathing.**
Record pulse and respiration rate immediately so you won't forget. Care plans are made based on your report.

9. **Before leaving resident, place call light within resident's reach.**
Allows resident to communicate with staff as necessary.

10. **Wash hands.**
Provides for infection control.

11. **Report any changes in resident to the nurse.**
Provides nurse with information to assess resident.

12. **Document procedure using facility guidelines.**
What you write is a legal record of what you did. If you don't document it, legally it didn't happen.

👁 *Your state testing company may divide taking the radial pulse and counting respirations into two separate procedures. In that case, you may need to explain what you are going to do before counting respirations. If so, that is for testing purposes only.*

Blood Pressure

Blood pressure is an important measure of health. Blood pressure is measured in millimeters of mercury (mmHg). The measurement shows how well the heart is working. There are two parts of blood pressure. They are the systolic measurement and diastolic measurement.

In the **systolic** phase, the heart is at work. It contracts and pushes blood from the left ventricle of the heart. The reading shows the pressure on the walls of arteries as blood is pumped through the body. The normal range for systolic blood pressure is 100–119 mmHg.

The second measurement reflects the **diastolic** phase. This is when the heart relaxes. The diastolic measurement is always lower than the systolic measurement. It shows the pressure in the arteries when the heart is at rest. The normal range for adults is 60–79 mmHg.

People with high blood pressure, or **hypertension**, have elevated systolic and/or diastolic blood pressures. A blood pressure level of 140/90 mmHg or higher is considered high. However, if blood pressure is between 120/80 mmHg and 139/89 mmHg, it is called prehypertension. This person does not have high blood pressure now but is likely to have it in the future. Report to the nurse if a resident's blood pressure is 140/90 or above.

Blood pressure is taken with a stethoscope and a blood pressure cuff, or sphygmomanometer (Fig. 6-20). There may be an electronic sphygmomanometer available. The systolic and diastolic pressure readings and pulse are displayed digitally. You do not need a stethoscope with an electronic sphygmomanometer.

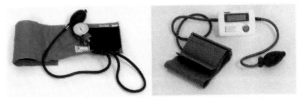

Fig. 6-20. a) A sphygmomanometer and b) an electronic sphygmomanometer.

When taking blood pressure, the first clear sound you will hear is the systolic pressure (top number). When the sound changes to a soft muffled thump or disappears, this is the diastolic pressure (bottom number). Blood pressure is recorded as a fraction. The sys-

6

Basic Nursing Skills

tolic reading is on top and the diastolic reading is on the bottom (for example: 120/80).

Never measure blood pressure on an arm that has an IV or any medical equipment. Avoid a side that has a cast, recent trauma, paralysis from a stroke, burn(s), or breast surgery (mastectomy).

This textbook includes two methods for taking blood pressure. They are the one-step method and the two-step method. In the two-step method, you will get an estimate of the systolic blood pressure before you start. After getting an estimated systolic reading, you will deflate the cuff and begin again. With the one-step method, you will not get an estimated systolic reading before getting the blood pressure reading. Your state may require that you know one or both of these methods. Follow your facility's policy on which method to use.

Taking and recording blood pressure (one-step method)

Equipment: sphygmomanometer (blood pressure cuff), stethoscope, alcohol wipes, pen and paper to record your findings

1. **Wash hands.**
   Provides for infection control.

2. **Identify yourself by name. Identify the resident by name.**
   Resident has right to know identity of his or her caregiver. Addressing resident by name shows respect and establishes correct identification.

3. **Explain procedure to the resident. Speak clearly, slowly, and directly. Maintain face-to-face contact whenever possible.**
   Promotes understanding and independence.

4. **Provide for resident's privacy with curtain, screen, or door.**
   Maintains resident's right to privacy and dignity.

5. **Position resident's arm with palm up. The arm should be level with the heart.**

A false low reading is possible if arm is above heart level.

6. **With the valve open, squeeze the cuff. Make sure it is completely deflated.**

7. **Place blood pressure cuff snugly on resident's upper arm. The center of the cuff is placed over the brachial artery (1-1½ inches above the elbow toward inside of elbow) (Fig. 6-21).**
   Cuff must be proper size and put on arm correctly so amount of pressure on artery is correct. If not, reading will be falsely high or low.

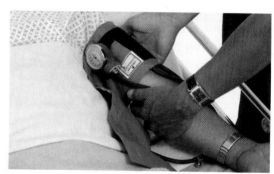

Fig. 6-21.

8. **Before using stethoscope, wipe diaphragm and earpieces with alcohol wipes.**
   Reduces pathogens, prevents ear infections and prevents spread of infection.

9. **Locate brachial pulse with fingertips.**

10. **Place diaphragm of stethoscope over brachial artery.**

11. **Place earpieces of stethoscope in ears.**

12. **Close the valve (clockwise) until it stops. Do not tighten it (Fig. 6-22).**
    Tight valves are too hard to release.

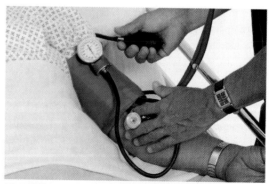

Fig. 6-22.

13. **Inflate cuff to 30 mmHg above the point at which the pulse is last heard or felt.**

14. **Open the valve slightly with thumb and index finger. Deflate cuff slowly.**
    Releasing the valve slowly allows you to hear beats accurately.

15. **Watch gauge. Listen for sound of pulse.**

16. **Remember the reading at which the first clear pulse sound is heard. This is the systolic pressure.**

17. **Continue listening for a change or muffling of pulse sound. The point of a change or the point the sound disappears is the diastolic pressure. Remember this reading.**

18. **Open the valve. Deflate cuff completely. Remove cuff.**
    An inflated cuff left on resident's arm can cause numbness and tingling. If you must take blood pressure again, completely deflate cuff and wait 30 seconds. Never partially deflate a cuff and then pump it up again. Blood vessels will be damaged and reading will be falsely high or low.

19. **Record both the systolic and diastolic pressures.**
    Record readings immediately so you won't forget. Care plans are made based on your report.

20. **Wipe diaphragm and earpieces of stethoscope with alcohol. Store equipment.**

21. **Before leaving, place call light within resident's reach. Remove privacy measures.**
    Allows resident to communicate with staff as necessary.

22. **Wash your hands.**
    Provides for infection control.

23. **Report any changes in resident to the nurse.**
    Provides nurse with information to assess resident.

24. **Document procedure using facility guidelines.**
    What you write is a legal record of what you did. If you don't document it, legally it didn't happen.

Taking and recording blood pressure (two-step method)

Equipment: sphygmomanometer (blood pressure cuff), stethoscope, alcohol wipes, pen and paper to record your findings

1. **Wash hands.**
   Provides for infection control.

2. **Identify yourself by name. Identify the resident by name.**
   Resident has right to know identity of his or her caregiver. Addressing resident by name shows respect and establishes correct identification.

3. **Explain procedure to resident. Speak clearly, slowly, and directly. Maintain face-to-face contact whenever possible.**
   Promotes understanding and independence.

4. **Provide for resident's privacy with curtain, screen, or door.**
   Maintains resident's right to privacy and dignity.

5. **Position resident's arm with palm up. The arm should be level with the heart.**
   A false low reading is possible if arm is above heart level.

6. **With the valve open, squeeze the cuff to make sure it is completely deflated.**

7. **Place blood pressure cuff snugly on resident's upper arm. The center of the cuff is placed over the brachial artery (1-1½ inches above the elbow toward inside of elbow).**
   Cuff must be proper size and put on arm correctly so amount of pressure on artery is correct. If not, reading will be falsely high or low.

8. **Locate the radial (wrist) pulse with fingertips.**

9. **Close the valve (clockwise) until it stops. Inflate cuff slowly, watching gauge.**
   If you inflate the cuff too quickly, you will not be able to identify the point where the pulse stops.

10. **Stop inflating when you can no longer feel the pulse. Note the reading. The number is an <u>estimate</u> of the systolic pressure.**

6

Basic Nursing Skills

This estimate helps you to not inflate the cuff too high later in this procedure. Inflating cuff too high is painful and may damage small blood vessels.

11. **Open the valve. Deflate cuff completely.**

    An inflated cuff left on resident's arm can cause numbness and tingling.

12. **Write down estimated systolic reading.**

13. **Before using stethoscope, wipe diaphragm and earpieces of stethoscope with alcohol wipes.**

    Reduces pathogens, prevents ear infections and prevents spread of infection.

14. **Locate brachial pulse with fingertips.**

15. **Place diaphragm of stethoscope over brachial artery.**

16. **Place earpieces of stethoscope in ears.**

17. **Close the valve (clockwise) until it stops. Do not tighten it.**

    Tight valves are too hard to release.

18. **Inflate cuff to 30 mmHg above your estimated systolic pressure.**

    Inflating cuff too high is painful and may damage small blood vessels.

19. **Open the valve slightly with thumb and index finger. Deflate cuff slowly.**

    Releasing the valve slowly allows you to hear beats accurately.

20. **Watch gauge. Listen for sound of pulse.**

21. **Remember the reading at which the first clear pulse sound is heard. This is the systolic pressure.**

22. **Continue listening for a change or muffling of pulse sound. The point of a change or the point the sound disappears is the diastolic pressure. Remember this reading.**

23. **Open the valve. Deflate cuff completely. Remove cuff.**

    An inflated cuff left on resident's arm can cause numbness and tingling. If you must take blood pressure again, completely deflate cuff and wait 30 seconds. Never partially deflate a cuff and then pump it up again. Blood vessels will be damaged and reading will be falsely high or low.

24. **Record systolic and diastolic pressures.**

    Record readings immediately so you won't forget. Care plans are made based on your report.

25. **Wipe diaphragm and earpieces of stethoscope with alcohol. Store equipment.**

26. **Before leaving, place call light within resident's reach. Remove privacy measures.**

    Allows resident to communicate with staff as necessary.

27. **Wash hands.**

    Provides for infection control.

28. **Report any changes in resident to the nurse.**

    Provides nurse with information to assess resident.

29. **Document procedure using facility guidelines.**

    What you write is a legal record of what you did. If you don't document it, legally it didn't happen.

Pain Management

It is important to observe and report on a resident's pain. Pain is called the "fifth vital sign" because it is so important to monitor.

Pain is uncomfortable. It is also a personal experience. It is different for each person. You spend the most time with residents. You play an important role in pain monitoring and prevention. Care plans are made based on your reports.

Pain is **not** a normal part of aging. Treat residents' complaints of pain seriously (Fig. 6-23). Listen to what residents are saying about the way they feel. Take action to help them. If a resident complains of pain, ask these questions to get the most accurate information. Immediately report the information to the nurse. Sustained pain may lead to withdrawal, depression, and isolation.

• Where is the pain?

- When did the pain start?
- Is the pain mild, moderate, or severe? To help find out, ask the resident to rate the pain on a scale of 1 to 10. Ten is the worst.
- Ask the resident to describe the pain. Make notes if you need to. Use the resident's words when reporting to the nurse.
- Ask the resident what he or she was doing before the pain started.
- Ask the resident how long the pain lasts and how often it occurs.
- Ask the resident what makes the pain better and what makes it feel worse.

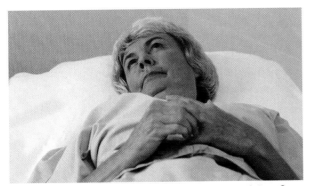

Fig. 6-23. Believe residents when they complain of pain. Being in pain is unpleasant. Help them by asking questions and reporting your observations.

Barriers to managing pain are:

- Fear of addiction to pain medication
- Feeling that pain is a normal part of aging
- Worrying about constipation and fatigue from pain medication
- Feeling that caregivers are too busy to deal with their pain
- Feeling that too much pain medication will cause death

Be patient and caring when helping residents who are in pain. If they are worried about the effects of pain medication or if they have questions about it, tell the nurse. Understand that some people do not feel comfortable saying that they are in pain. A

person's culture affects how he or she responds to pain. Some cultures believe that it is best not to react to pain. Other cultures believe in expressing pain freely. Watch for body language or other messages that residents may be in pain. Signs and symptoms of pain to observe and report are:

Observing and Reporting
Pain

Report any of these to the nurse:

- increased pulse, respirations, blood pressure
- sweating
- nausea
- vomiting
- tightening the jaw
- squeezing eyes shut
- holding a body part tightly
- frowning
- grinding teeth
- increased restlessness
- agitation or tension
- change in behavior
- crying
- sighing
- groaning
- breathing heavily
- difficulty moving or walking

Measures to reduce pain are:

- Report complaints of pain or unrelieved pain promptly to the nurse.
- Gently position the body in good alignment. Use pillows for support. Help in changes of position if the resident wishes.
- Give back rubs.
- Offer warm baths or showers.

6

Basic Nursing Skills

• Help the resident to the bathroom or com-mode or offer the bedpan or urinal.

• Encourage slow, deep breaths when the resident has trouble breathing.

• Provide a calm and quiet environment. Use soft music to distract the resident.

• Always be patient, caring, gentle, and sympathetic.

• Note the resident's emotional response to pain and how the resident coped with the pain.

Unit 3. Explain how to measure height and weight

You will check residents' weights and heights as part of your care. Height is checked less often than weight. Weight changes can be signs of illness. You must report **any** weight loss or gain, no matter how small.

Measuring and recording weight of an ambulatory resident

Equipment: standing scale, pen and paper to record your findings

1. **Wash hands.**
   Provides for infection control.

2. **Identify yourself by name. Identify the resident by name.**
   Resident has right to know identity of his or her caregiver. Addressing resident by name shows respect and establishes correct identification.

3. **Explain procedure to resident. Speak clearly, slowly, and directly. Maintain face-to-face contact whenever possible.**
   Promotes understanding and independence.

4. **Provide for resident's privacy with curtain, screen, or door.**
   Maintains resident's right to privacy and dignity.

5. **Start with scale balanced at zero before weighing resident.**
   Scale must be balanced on zero for weight to be accurate.

6. **Help resident to step onto the center of the scale.**

7. **Determine resident's weight. This is done by balancing the scale. Make the balance bar level. Move the small and large weight indicators until the bar balances (Fig. 6-24). Add these two numbers together.**

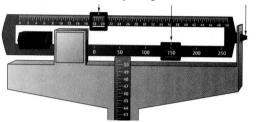

Small Weight Indicator   Large Weight Indicator   Balance Bar

Fig. 6-24.

8. **Assist resident off scale before recording weight.**
   Protects against falls.

9. **Record weight.**
   Record weight immediately so you won't forget. Care plans are made based on your report.

10. **Remove privacy measures.**

11. **Before leaving, place call light within resident's reach.**
    Allows resident to communicate with staff as necessary.

12. **Wash hands.**
    Provides for infection control.

13. **Report any changes in resident to the nurse.**
    Provides nurse with information to assess resident.

14. **Document procedure using facility guidelines.**
    What you write is a legal record of what you did. If you don't document it, legally it didn't happen.

Some residents will not be able to get out of a wheelchair easily. These residents may be weighed on a wheelchair scale. With this scale, wheelchairs are rolled onto the scale (Fig. 6-25). On some wheelchair scales, you will need to subtract the weight of the wheelchair from a resident's weight. In this case, weigh the empty wheelchair first. Then subtract the wheelchair's weight from the total. Some wheelchairs are marked with their weight.

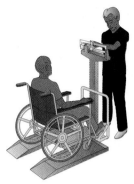

Fig. 6-25. A type of wheelchair scale.

Some residents will not be able to get out of bed. Weighing these residents requires a special scale (Fig. 6-26). Before using a bed scale, know how to use it properly and safely. Follow your facility's procedure and any manufacturer's instructions.

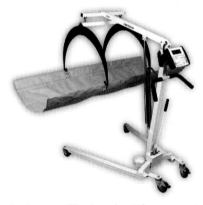

Fig. 6-26. A type of bed scale. (Photo courtesy of Detecto, www.detecto.com, 800-641-2008)

Measuring and recording height of an ambulatory resident

Equipment: standing scale, pen and paper to record your findings

1. **Wash hands.**
   Provides for infection control.

2. **Identify yourself by name. Identify the resident by name.**
   Resident has right to know identity of his or her caregiver. Addressing resident by name shows respect and establishes correct identification.

3. **Explain procedure to resident. Speak clearly, slowly, and directly. Maintain face-to-face contact whenever possible.**
   Promotes understanding and independence.

4. **Provide for resident's privacy with curtain, screen, or door.**
   Maintains resident's right to privacy and dignity.

5. **Help resident to step onto scale, facing away from the scale.**

6. **Ask resident to stand straight. Help as needed.**
   Ensures accurate reading.

7. **Pull up measuring rod from back of scale. Gently lower measuring rod until it rests flat on resident's head (Fig. 6-27).**

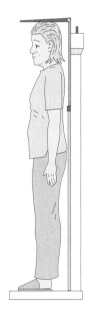

Fig. 6-27.

8. **Determine resident's height.**

9. **Help resident off scale before recording height. Make sure measuring rod does not hit resident in the head while trying to help resident off the scale.**

10. **Record height.**
    Record height immediately so you won't forget. Care plans are made based on your report.

11. **Before leaving, place call light within resident's reach. Remove privacy measures.**
    Allows resident to communicate with staff as necessary.

6

Basic Nursing Skills

12. **Wash hands.**

Provides for infection control.

13. **Report any changes in resident to the nurse.**

Provides nurse with information to assess resident.

14. **Document procedure according to facility guidelines.**

What you write is a legal record of what you did. If you don't document it, legally it didn't happen.

The rod measures height in inches and fractions of inches. Record the total number of inches. If you have to change inches into feet, remember that there are 12 inches in a foot.

If resident cannot get out of bed, measure height with a tape measure (Fig. 6-28). Position the resident lying straight in bed. Mark the sheet with a pencil at the top of the head and at the bottom of the feet (Fig. 6-29). Measure the distance between the marks. Record the height.

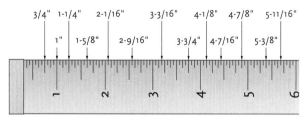

Fig. 6-28. A tape measure.

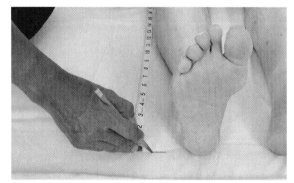

Fig. 6-29. Make marks on the sheet at the resident's head and feet.

If the resident cannot lie in a straight position due to contractures, a tape measure can

still be used to measure height. Start at the top of the head. Continue to the base of the heel, following the curves of the spine and legs. Total the number of inches and record them. Note that the resident has contractures when recording this height.

Unit 4. Explain restraints and how to promote a restraint-free environment

A **restraint** is a physical or chemical way to restrict voluntary movement or behavior. Common physical restraints are the vest restraint, belt restraint, wrist/ankle restraint, and the mitt restraint. Physical restraints are also called postural supports or protective devices. Side rails and special chairs, such as geriatric chairs, are also physical restraints (Figs. 6-30 and 6-31). Chemical restraints are medications given to control behavior.

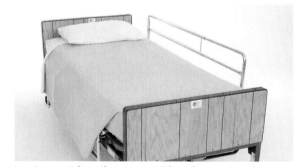

Fig. 6-30. Side rails are considered restraints because they restrict movement.

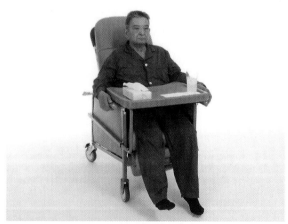

Fig. 6-31. When the tray table is attached, a geriatric chair, or geri-chair, is considered a restraint.

In the past, restraints were commonly ordered for these reasons:

- To keep a person from injuring self or others
- To keep a person from pulling out tubing that is needed for treatment
- To keep a person with dementia or who is confused from wandering
- To prevent falls

Restraint usage was abused by caregivers. The abuse led to new restrictions and laws on their use. Today, the use of both physical and chemical restraints in facilities has greatly decreased.

Generally, restraints are only used as a last resort. **Restraints can never be used without a doctor's order**. It is against the law for staff to use restraints for convenience or discipline.

There are many problems with restraints. Some negative effects of restraint use are:

- reduced blood circulation
- stress on the heart
- incontinence
- constipation
- weakened muscles and bones
- loss of bone mass
- muscle atrophy (weakening or wasting of the muscle)
- pressure sores
- risk of suffocation
- pneumonia
- less activity, leading to poor appetite
- sleep disorders
- loss of dignity
- loss of independence
- increased agitation
- increased depression and/or withdrawal
- poor self-esteem

Restraints have also caused severe injury and even death.

Laws allow the use of restraints only when absolutely necessary for the safety of the person, others around that person, and staff. State and federal agencies encourage facilities to take steps toward a restraint-free environment. **Restraint-free** care means that restraints are not used for any reason. They are usually not kept by the facility. To reach this goal, many nursing homes use creative ideas called **restraint alternatives**. A restraint alternative is any intervention used in the place of a restraint or that reduces the need for a restraint. Examples of restraint alternatives include:

- Improve safety measures to prevent accidents and falls. Improve lighting.
- Use postural devices to support and protect the residents' bodies.
- Make sure call light is within reach. Answer call lights promptly.
- Ambulate the resident when he or she is restless. Add exercise into the care plan. Provide activities for those who wander at night.
- Encourage activities and independence. Escort the person to social activities. Increase visits and social interaction.
- Give frequent help with toileting. Help with cleaning immediately after an episode of incontinence.
- Bed or body alarms can be used in place of side rails. They can also be used with wheelchairs or chairs. They help prevent falls by alerting staff when residents attempt to leave the bed or chair. Alarms can also be used for confused residents who wander. If a resident is ordered to have a body alarm (bed or chair), make sure it is on the resident and turned on.

6

Basic Nursing Skills

6

Basic Nursing Skills

- Offer food or drink. Offer reading materials.

- Distract or redirect interest. Give the person a repetitive task.

- Decrease the noise level. Listen to soothing music. Use massage or relaxation techniques.

- Assess medications. Reduce pain by scheduling medications. Report pain to the nurse.

- Offer a few minutes of one-on-one time with a caregiver. Provide familiar caregivers. Increase the number of caregivers with family and volunteers.

- Use a team approach to meeting needs.

- Offer training to teach gentle approaches to difficult people.

There are also several types of pads, belts, special chairs, and alarms that can be used instead of restraints (Fig. 6-32).

A restrained resident must be monitored constantly. The resident must be checked every 15 minutes. At least every two hours the following must be done:

- Release the restraint for at least ten minutes.

- Offer assistance with toileting. Check for episodes of incontinence. Provide incontinence care.

- Offer fluids.

- Check skin for irritation. Report any red areas to the nurse immediately.

- Reposition the resident.

- Ambulate resident if able.

If you are asked to apply a restraint, follow the manufacturer's instructions.

The survey team will look for evidence that the facility is protecting a resident's right to be free from restraints. When a restraint is necessary, the team will look to see that staff protect the resident from harm.

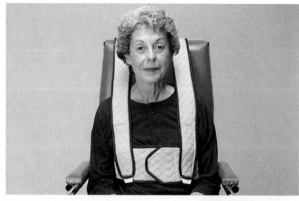
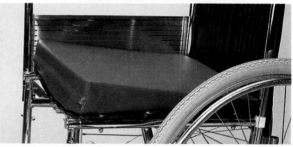
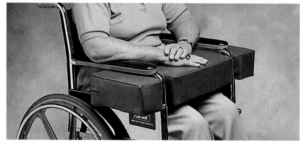

Fig. 6-32. a) A Posey Torso Support, b) A Posey Deluxe Wedge Cushion, c) A lap top cushion. (Photos courtesy of North Coast Medical, Inc., www.ncmedical.com, 800-821-9319.)

Unit 5. Define fluid balance and explain intake and output (I&O)

To maintain health, the body must take in a certain amount of fluid each day. Fluid comes in the form of liquids you drink. It is also found in semi-liquid foods like gelatin, soup, ice cream, pudding, and yogurt. The fluid a person consumes is called **intake**, or input. All fluid taken in each day cannot stay in the body. It must be eliminated as **output**. Output includes urine, feces, and vomitus. It also includes perspiration and moisture in the air we exhale.

Fluid balance is maintaining equal intake and output, or taking in and eliminating equal amounts of fluids. Some residents must have their intake and output, or I&O, watched and recorded. You will need to measure and document all the fluids the resident takes by mouth. You will also need to measure and record all urine and vomitus. This is recorded on an Intake/Output (I&O) sheet (Fig. 6-33). (See chapter 7 for more information on fluid balance.)

INTAKE AND OUTPUT RECORD

DATE	SHIFT	INTAKE (IN CC'S) ORAL	OUTPUT (IN CC'S) VOIDED	CATHETER	NUMBER OF INCONTINENT EPISODES (IF APPLICABLE)	DATE	SHIFT	INTAKE (IN CC'S) ORAL	OUTPUT (IN CC'S) VOIDED	CATHETER	NUMBER OF INCONTINENT EPISODES (IF APPLICABLE)
	7-3						7-3				
	3-11						3-11				
	11-7						11-7				
	24 HR. TOTAL						24 HR. TOTAL				
	7-3						7-3				
	3-11						3-11				
	11-7						11-7				
	24 HR. TOTAL						24 HR. TOTAL				
	7-3						7-3				
	3-11						3-11				
	11-7						11-7				
	24 HR. TOTAL						24 HR. TOTAL				
	7-3						7-3				
	3-11						3-11				
	11-7						11-7				
	24 HR. TOTAL						24 HR. TOTAL				
	7-3						7-3				
	3-11						3-11				
	11-7						11-7				
	24 HR. TOTAL						24 HR. TOTAL				
	7-3						7-3				
	3-11						3-11				
	11-7						11-7				
	24 HR. TOTAL						24 HR. TOTAL				
	7-3						7-3				
	3-11						3-11				
	11-7						11-7				
	24 HR. TOTAL						24 HR. TOTAL				

NAME-Last	First	Middle	Attending Physician	Record No.	Room/Bed

INTAKE AND OUTPUT RECORD

Fig. 6-33. A sample intake and output (I&O) form.

Conversions

A cubic centimeter (cc) is a unit of measure equal to 1 milliliter (ml). Follow your facility's policies on whether to document using "cc" or "ml."

1 oz. = 30 cc or 30 ml

2 oz. = 60 cc

3 oz. = 90 cc

4 oz. = 120 cc

5 oz. = 150 cc

6 oz. = 180 cc

7 oz. = 210 cc

8 oz. = 240 cc

¼ cup = 2 oz. = 60 cc

½ cup = 4 oz. = 120 cc

1 cup = 8 oz. = 240 cc

Measuring and recording urinary output

Equipment: I&O sheet, graduate (measuring container), gloves, pen and paper to record your findings

1. **Wash hands.**
    Provides for infection control.

2. **Put on gloves before handling bedpan/urinal.**

3. **Pour the contents of the bedpan or urinal into measuring container. Do not spill or splash any of the urine.**

4. **Measure the amount of urine. Keep container level (Fig. 6-34).**
    Helps get accurate reading.

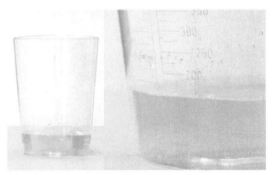

Fig. 6-34. A graduate is a measuring container.

5. **After measuring urine, empty measuring container into toilet. Do not splash.**
    Reduces risk of contamination.

6. **Rinse measuring container. Pour rinse water into toilet. Clean container using facility guidelines.**

7. **Rinse bedpan/urinal. Pour rinse water into toilet. Use disinfectant if ordered.**

8. **Return bedpan/urinal and measuring container to proper storage.**

9. **Remove and dispose of gloves.**

10. **Wash hands before recording output.**
    Provides for infection control.

11. **Record contents of container in output column on sheet.**

    Record amount immediately so you won't forget. Care plans are made based on your report. What you write is a legal record of what you did. If you don't document it, legally it didn't happen.

12. **Report any changes in resident to the nurse.**

    Provides nurse with information to assess resident.

Catheter Care

A **catheter** is a tube used to drain urine from the bladder. A **straight catheter** does not stay inside the person. It is removed immediately after the urine is drained. An **indwelling catheter** remains inside the bladder for a period of time (Figs. 6-35 and 6-36). The urine drains into a bag. NAs do not usually insert, remove, or irrigate catheters. You may be asked to provide daily care for the catheter, cleaning the area around the urethral opening, and emptying the drainage bag.

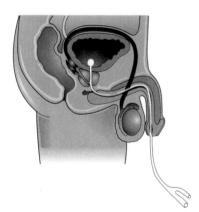

Fig. 6-35. An indwelling catheter (male).

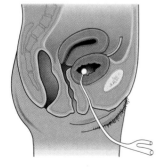

Fig. 6-36. An indwelling catheter (female).

An external, or **condom catheter** (also called a Texas catheter), has an attachment on the end that fits onto the penis. The attachment is fastened with tape. The external catheter is changed daily or as needed. Unit 6 has information on other kinds of tubing.

Guidelines
Catheters

- Always make sure that the drainage bag is lower than the hips or bladder. Urine must never flow from the bag or tubing back into the bladder. This can cause infection.

- Keep the drainage bag off the floor.

- Tubing should be kept as straight as possible. It should not be kinked.

- The genital area must be kept clean to prevent infection.

Observing and Reporting
Catheter Care

- blood in the urine or any other unusual appearance

- catheter bag does not fill after several hours

- catheter bag fills suddenly

- catheter is not in place

- urine leaks from the catheter

- resident reports pain or pressure

- odor

Providing catheter care

Equipment: bath blanket, protective pad, bath basin, soap, bath thermometer, 2-4 washcloths or wipes, 1 towel, gloves

1. **Wash hands.**

   Provides for infection control.

2. **Identify yourself by name. Identify the resident by name.**

   Resident has right to know identity of his or her caregiver. Addressing resident by name shows respect and establishes correct identification.

3. **Explain procedure to resident. Speak clearly, slowly, and directly. Maintain face-to-face contact whenever possible.**
Promotes understanding and independence.

4. **Provide for resident's privacy with curtain, screen, or door.**
Maintains resident's right to privacy and dignity.

5. **Adjust bed to a safe working level, usually waist high. Lock bed wheels.**
Prevents injury to you and to resident.

6. **Lower head of bed. Position resident lying flat on her back.**

7. **Remove or fold back top bedding. Keep resident covered with bath blanket.**
Promotes resident's privacy.

8. **Test water temperature with thermometer or your wrist and ensure it is safe. Water temperature should be 105° to 109° F. Have resident check water temperature. Adjust if necessary.**
Resident's sense of touch may be different than yours; therefore, resident is best able to identify a comfortable water temperature.

9. **Put on gloves.**
Prevents you from coming into contact with body fluids.

10. **Ask the resident to flex her knees and raise the buttocks off the bed by pushing against the mattress with her feet. Place clean protective pad under her buttocks.**
Keeps linen from getting wet.

11. **Expose only the area necessary to clean the catheter.**
Promotes resident's privacy.

12. **Place towel or pad under catheter tubing before washing.**
Helps keep linen from getting wet.

13. **Apply soap to wet washcloth. Clean area around meatus. Use a clean area of the washcloth for each stroke.**

14. **Hold catheter near meatus. Avoid tugging the catheter.**

15. **Clean at least four inches of catheter nearest meatus. Move in only one direction, away from meatus. Use a clean area of the cloth for each stroke.**
Prevents infection.

16. **Rinse area around meatus, using a clean area of washcloth for each stroke.**

17. **Rinse at least four inches of catheter nearest meatus. Move in only one direction, away from meatus (Fig. 6-37). Use a clean area of the cloth for each stroke.**

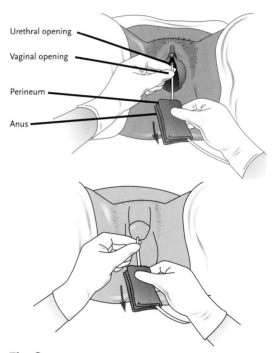

Urethral opening
Vaginal opening
Perineum
Anus

Fig. 6-37.

18. **Remove towel or pad from under catheter tubing.**

19. **Replace top covers. Remove bath blanket.**

20. **Dispose of linen in proper containers.**

21. **Empty, rinse, and wipe basin. Return to proper storage.**

22. **Remove and dispose of gloves.**

23. **Return bed to proper level. Remove privacy measures.**
Lowering the bed provides for safety.

24. **Before leaving, place call light within resident's reach.**
Allows resident to communicate with staff as needed.

25. **Wash hands.**

    Provides for infection control.

26. **Report any changes in resident to the nurse.**

    Provides nurse with information to assess resident.

27. **Document procedure using facility guidelines.**

    What you write is a legal record of what you did. If you don't document it, legally it didn't happen.

👁 *When cleaning the catheter, move in one direction only, away from the genital area. Use a clean area of the cloth for each stroke.*

Collecting Specimens

You may be asked to collect a specimen from a resident. A **specimen** is a sample. Different types of specimens are used for different tests. You may be asked to collect these different types of specimens:

- Urine (routine, clean catch/mid-stream, or 24-hour)

- Stool (feces)

Sputum specimens are collected to check for respiratory problems. **Sputum** is mucus coughed up from the lungs. Early morning is the best time to collect sputum.

A plastic collection container called a "hat" is sometimes put into a toilet to collect and measure urine and stool (Fig. 6-38). Hats should be labeled. They must be cleaned after each use.

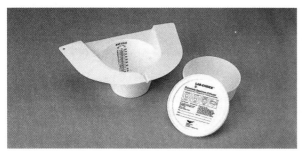

Fig. 6-38. A "hat" is placed under the toilet seat to collect specimens.

Some residents will be able to collect their own specimens. Others will need your help. Be sure to explain exactly how the specimen must be collected.

Collecting a routine urine specimen

Equipment: urine specimen container and lid, label, gloves, bedpan or urinal (if resident cannot get to the bathroom), "hat" for toilet (if resident can get to the bathroom), 2 plastic bags, washcloth, towel, paper towel, supplies for perineal care, pen

1. **Wash hands.**

   Provides for infection control.

2. **Identify yourself by name. Identify the resident by name.**

   Resident has right to know identity of his or her caregiver. Addressing resident by name shows respect and establishes correct identification.

3. **Explain procedure to the resident. Speak clearly, slowly, and directly. Maintain face-to-face contact whenever possible.**

   Promotes understanding and independence.

4. **Provide for resident's privacy with curtain, screen, or door.**

   Maintains resident's right to privacy and dignity.

5. **Put on gloves.**

   Prevents you from coming into contact with body fluids.

6. **Help the resident to the bathroom or commode, or offer the bedpan or urinal.**

7. **Have resident void into "hat," urinal, or bedpan. Ask the resident not to put toilet paper in with the sample. Provide a plastic bag to discard toilet paper.**

   Paper ruins the sample.

8. **After urination, help as necessary with perineal care. Help resident wash his or her hands. Make the resident comfortable.**

9. **Take bedpan, urinal, or commode pail to the bathroom.**

10. **Pour urine into the specimen container.**

Specimen container should be at least half full.

11. Cover the urine container with its lid. Do not touch the inside of container. Wipe off the outside with a paper towel.
Prevents contamination.

12. Place the container in a plastic bag.
Provides for safe transport.

13. If using a bedpan or urinal, discard extra urine. Rinse and clean equipment. Use approved disinfectant if facility policy. Store.

14. Remove and dispose of gloves. Wash hands.
Provides for infection control.

15. Complete the label for the container. Write the resident's name, room number, the date, and time.

16. Make resident comfortable.

17. Return bed to appropriate position if adjusted. Remove privacy measures.

18. Before leaving, place call light within resident's reach.
Allows resident to communicate with staff as necessary.

19. Wash hands.
Provides for infection control.

20. Report any changes in resident to the nurse.
Provides nurse with information to assess resident.

21. Document procedure using facility guidelines. Note amount and characteristics of urine.
What you write is a legal record of what you did. If you don't document it, legally it didn't happen.

Collecting a clean catch (mid-stream) urine specimen

Equipment: specimen kit with container, label, cleaning solution, gauze or towelettes, gloves, bedpan or urinal if resident cannot use the bathroom, plastic bag, washcloth, paper towel, towel, supplies for perineal care, pen

The specimen is called **mid-stream** because the first and last urine are not included in the sample.

1. Wash hands.
Provides for infection control.

2. Identify yourself to resident by name. Identify the resident by name.
Resident has right to know identity of his or her caregiver. Addressing resident by name shows respect and establishes correct identification.

3. Explain procedure to resident. Speak clearly, slowly, and directly. Maintain face-to-face contact whenever possible.
Promotes understanding and independence.

4. Provide for resident's privacy with curtain, screen, or door.
Maintains resident's right to privacy and dignity.

5. Put on gloves.
Prevents you from coming into contact with body fluids.

6. Open the specimen kit. Do not touch the inside of the container or lid.
Prevents contamination.

7. If the resident cannot clean his or her perineal area, you will do it. Using the towelettes or g`auze and cleansing solution, clean the area around the meatus. For females, separate the labia. Wipe from front to back along one side. Discard towelette/gauze. With a new towelette or gauze, wipe from front to back along the other side. Using a new towelette or gauze, wipe down the middle.

For males, clean the head of the penis. Use circular motions with the towelettes or gauze. Clean thoroughly. Change towelettes/gauze after each circular motion. Discard after use. If the man is uncircumcised, pull back the foreskin of the penis before cleaning. Hold it back during urination. Make sure it is pulled back down after collecting the specimen.

Improper cleaning can infect urinary tract and contaminate the sample.

8. **Ask the resident to urinate into the bedpan, urinal, or toilet, and to stop before urination is complete.**

9. **Place the container under the urine stream. Have the resident start urinating again. Fill the container at least half full. Have the resident finish urinating in bedpan, urinal, or toilet.**

10. **Cover the urine container with its lid. Do not touch the inside of the container. Wipe off the outside with a paper towel.**

11. **Place the container in a plastic bag.**
    Provides for safe transport.

12. **If using a bedpan or urinal, discard extra urine. Rinse and clean equipment. Use approved disinfectant if facility policy. Store.**

13. **Remove and dispose of gloves. Wash hands. Help resident wash his hands.**
    Promotes infection control.

14. **Complete the label for the container. Write the resident's name, address, the date, and time.**

15. **Make resident comfortable.**

16. **Return bed to appropriate position if adjusted. Remove privacy measures.**

17. **Before leaving, place call light within resident's reach.**
    Allows resident to communicate with staff as necessary.

18. **Wash hands.**
    Provides for infection control.

19. **Report any changes in resident to the nurse.**
    Provides nurse with information to assess resident.

20. **Document procedure using facility guidelines. Note amount and characteristics of urine.**
    What you write is a legal record of what you did. If you don't document it, legally it didn't happen.

Collecting a stool specimen

Equipment: specimen container and lid, 2 tongue blades, 2 pairs of gloves, bedpan if resident cannot use the bathroom or commode, specimen pan if resident uses toilet or commode, 2 plastic bags, toilet tissue, laboratory slip, washcloth or towel, supplies for perineal care, pen

Ask the resident to let you know when he or she can have a bowel movement. Be ready to collect the specimen.

1. **Wash hands.**
   Provides for infection control.

2. **Identify yourself to resident by name. Identify the resident by name.**
   Resident has right to know identity of his or her caregiver. Addressing resident by name shows respect and establishes correct identification.

3. **Explain procedure to resident. Speak clearly, slowly, and directly. Maintain face-to-face contact whenever possible.**
   Promotes understanding and independence.

4. **Provide for resident's privacy with curtain, screen, or door.**
   Maintains resident's right to privacy and dignity.

5. **Put on gloves.**
   Prevents you from coming into contact with body fluids.

6. **When the resident is ready to move bowels, ask him not to urinate at the same time. Ask him not to put toilet paper in with the sample. Provide a plastic bag for toilet paper.**
   Urine and paper ruin the sample.

7. **Fit specimen pan to toilet or commode, or provide resident with bedpan. Leave the room. Ask the resident to signal when he is finished with the bowel movement. Make sure call light is within reach.**
   Promotes resident's privacy and dignity.

8. **After the bowel movement, help as necessary with perineal care. Help resident wash his or her hands. Make the resident comfortable. Remove gloves.**

9. Wash hands again.

10. Put on clean gloves.

11. Using the two tongue blades, take about two tablespoons of stool and put it in the container. Cover it tightly.

12. Wrap the tongue blades in toilet paper and throw them away. Empty the bedpan or container into the toilet. Clean equipment. Use approved disinfectant if facility policy. Store.

13. Label the container with the resident's name, address, the date, and time. Bag the specimen.

14. Remove and dispose of gloves.

15. Make resident comfortable.

16. Return bed to appropriate position if adjusted. Remove privacy measures.

17. Before leaving, place call light within resident's reach.

    Allows resident to communicate with staff as necessary.

18. Wash hands.

    Provides for infection control.

19. Report any changes in resident to the nurse.

    Provides nurse with information to assess resident.

20. Document procedure using facility guidelines. Note amount and characteristics of stool.

    What you write is a legal record of what you did. If you don't document it, legally it didn't happen.

Unit 6. Explain care guidelines for different types of tubing

Residents with breathing difficulties may receive oxygen. It is more concentrated than what is in the air. Oxygen is prescribed by a doctor. Nursing assistants never stop, adjust, or administer oxygen. Oxygen may be piped into a resident's room through a central system. It may be in tanks or produced by an oxygen concentrator. An oxygen concentrator changes air in the room into air with more oxygen.

Oxygen is a very dangerous fire hazard because it makes other things burn. Oxygen itself does not burn. It merely supports combustion. **Combustion** means the process of burning. Working around oxygen requires special safety precautions.

Guidelines
Working Safely Around Oxygen Equipment

- Remove all fire hazards from the room or area. Fire hazards include electric shavers, hair dryers, or other electrical appliances (Fig. 6-39). They also include flammable liquids. **Flammable** means easily ignited and capable of burning quickly. Examples of flammable liquids are alcohol and nail polish remover.

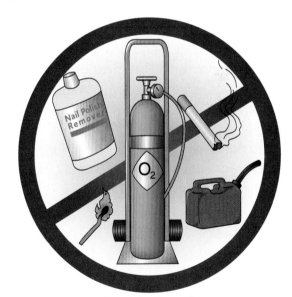

Fig. 6-39. Examples of fire hazards.

- Tell the nurse of fire hazards residents do not want removed.

- Post "No Smoking" and "Oxygen in Use" signs. Never allow smoking where oxygen is used or stored.

- Never allow candles or other open flames around oxygen.

6

Basic Nursing Skills

- Learn how to turn oxygen off in case of fire if facility allows this. Never adjust the oxygen level.

- Report if the nasal cannula or face mask causes irritation. Check behind ears for irritation from tubing (Fig. 6-40).

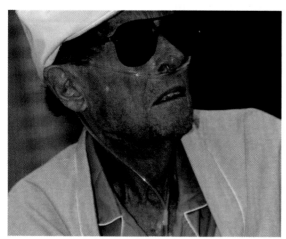

Fig. 6-40. A resident with a nasal cannula.

IV stands for **intravenous**, or into a vein. A resident with an IV receives medication, nutrition, or fluids through a vein. When a doctor prescribes an IV, a nurse inserts a needle or tube into a vein. This gives direct access to the bloodstream. Medication, nutrition, or fluids either drip from a bag suspended on a pole or are pumped by a portable pump through a tube and into the vein (Fig. 6-41). Some residents with chronic conditions have a permanent opening for IVs. It has been surgically created to allow easy access for IV fluids.

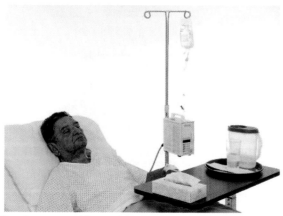

Fig. 6-41. A resident with an IV.

Nursing assistants never insert or remove IV lines. You will not be responsible for care of the IV site. Your only responsibility for IV care is to report and document any observations of changes or problems with the IV.

Observing and Reporting IVs

Report any of the following to the nurse:

- The tube/needle falls out or is removed.

- The tubing disconnects.

- The dressing around the IV site is loose or not intact.

- Blood is in the tubing or around the site of the IV.

- The site is swollen or discolored.

- The resident reports pain.

- The bag is broken, or the level of fluid does not seem to decrease.

- The IV fluid is not dripping.

- The IV fluid is nearly gone.

- The pump beeps, indicating a problem.

Do not do any of these when caring for a resident with an IV:

- take a blood pressure reading on an arm with an IV

- get the IV site wet

- pull or catch the tubing in anything, such as clothing

- leave the tubing kinked

- lower the IV bag below the IV site

- touch the clamp

- disconnect the IV from pump or turn off alarm

See chapter 5 for guidelines on how to apply a gown on a resident with an IV. See chapter 7 for information on gastric tubes.

Unit 7. **Discuss a resident's unit and related care**

A resident's unit is the room or area where the resident lives. It contains furniture and personal items. The unit is the resident's home. It must be treated with respect. Always knock and wait for permission before entering. Once personal items are in place within a room or unit, do not move them without permission. If a safety hazard exists, inform the nurse. He or she will handle the situation.

Each unit may have slightly different equipment. Standard unit equipment includes:

- Bed
- Bedside stand
- Overbed table
- Chair
- Emesis basin
- Bedpan
- Urinal
- Bath basin
- Call light
- Privacy curtain

Residents can store small items in bedside stands. The water pitcher and cup are often placed on top of the bedside stand. A telephone and/or a radio and other items, such as photos, may also be placed there.

The overbed table may be used for meals or personal care. It is a clean area. It must be kept clean and free of clutter. Bedpans and urinals and soiled linen should not be placed on overbed tables.

The intercom system is the most common call system. When the resident presses the button, a light will be seen and/or a bell will be heard at the nurses' station. The call light allows the resident to contact staff anytime. It is important to always place the call light within the resident's reach. Answer all call lights immediately.

You will be taught the right way to use many pieces of equipment. Know how to use and care for all equipment. This prevents infection and injury. If you do not know how to use a piece of equipment, ask for help.

Guidelines
Resident's Unit

- Clean the overbed table after use. Place it within the resident's reach before leaving.

- Keep the call light within the resident's reach at all times. Check to see that the resident can reach the call light every time you leave the room.

- Remove crumbs from the bed right after meals. Straighten bed linens as needed.

- Before leaving a resident's room, re-stock supplies. This includes facial tissues, bathroom tissue, paper towels, soap, or any other needed item.

- Check equipment daily. Make sure it is working properly and not damaged. If you find any damaged equipment, such as frayed or cracked cords, report it to the nurse or appropriate department.

- Refill water pitchers regularly unless resident has a fluid restriction. Promptly report to a nurse if a resident is not drinking his fluids.

- Remove anything that might cause odors or safety hazards, like trash, clutter or spills. Clean up spills promptly. Throw out disposable supplies. Empty trash at least once per shift. Replace any equipment that is stained or has an odor.

- Report signs of insects or pests right away.

6

Basic Nursing Skills

- Do not move resident's belongings. Do not discard resident's items. Respect the resident's things.

After providing care, tidy the area. Clean and put away equipment. Providing a clean, safe, and orderly environment is part of your job.

Unit 8. Explain the importance of sleep and perform proper bedmaking

Sleep and rest are two basic needs that must be met. Sleep provides us with new cells and energy. Many elderly persons, especially those who are living away from their homes, have sleep problems. Many things can affect sleep. Fear, anxiety, noise, diet, medications, and illness all affect sleep. Sharing a room with another person can disturb sleeping. When a resident complains of lack of sleep, staff should observe for:

- sleeping too much during the day
- too much caffeine late in the day
- dressing in night clothes during day instead of daytime wear
- eating too late at night
- refusing medication ordered for sleep
- taking new medications
- TV or light on late at night
- pain

Lack of sleep causes many problems. These include decreased mental function, reduced reaction time, and irritability. Sleep deprivation also decreases immune system function.

Bedmaking

Some residents spend much or all of their time in bed. Careful bedmaking is essential for comfort, cleanliness, and health. Linens should always be changed after personal care, such as bed baths. Change them any time bedding or sheets are damp, soiled, or in need of straightening. Bed linens should be changed often for three reasons:

1. Sheets that are damp, wrinkled, or bunched up are uncomfortable. They may keep the resident from sleeping well.

2. Microorganisms live in moist, warm environments. Bedding that is damp or unclean may cause infection and disease.

3. Residents who spend long hours in bed are at risk for pressure sores. Sheets that do not lie flat increase this risk by cutting off circulation.

Guidelines
Bedmaking

- Before getting clean linen, wash your hands.

- When collecting bed linen, carry it away from you. If linen touches your uniform, it is contaminated (Fig. 6-42).

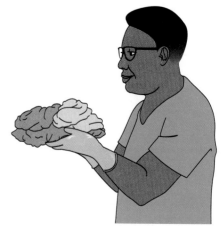

Fig. 6-42. Carry dirty linen away from your uniform.

- Do not shake linen. It may spread airborne contaminants.

- Do not take linen from one resident's room to another resident's room. This can spread pathogens.

- When removing dirty linen, roll it away from you.

- Wear gloves when removing linens.

- Look for personal items, such as dentures, hearing aids, jewelry, and glasses, before removing linens.

- Change linens when wet, soiled, or too wrinkled for comfort. Residents can develop pressure sores if left on wet, soiled, or wrinkled linen.

- Keep beds smooth and wrinkle- and crumb-free. Lumps, crumbs, and wrinkles irritate skin and cause pressure sores.

- Change disposable pads whenever they become soiled or wet. Dispose of them properly.

If a resident cannot get out of bed, you must change the linens with the resident in bed. An **occupied bed** is a bed made while the resident is in the bed. When making the bed, use a wide stance. Bend your knees. Avoid bending from the waist, especially when tucking sheets or blankets under the mattress. Mattresses can be heavy. Bend your knees to avoid injury. It is easier to make an empty bed than one with a resident in it. An **unoccupied bed** is a bed made while no resident is in the bed. If the resident can be moved, your job will be easier.

Making an occupied bed

Equipment: clean linen: mattress pad, fitted or flat bottom sheet, waterproof bed protector if needed, cotton draw sheet, flat top sheet, blanket(s), bath blanket, pillowcase(s), gloves

1. **Wash hands.**
   Provides for infection control.

2. **Identify yourself by name. Identify the resident by name.**
   Resident has right to know identity of his or her caregiver. Addressing resident by name shows respect and establishes correct identification.

3. **Explain procedure to resident. Speak clearly, slowly, and directly. Maintain face-to-face contact whenever possible.**
   Promotes understanding and independence.

4. **Provide for resident's privacy with curtain, screen, or door.**
   Maintains resident's right to privacy and dignity.

5. **Place clean linen on clean surface within reach (e.g., bedside stand, overbed table, or chair).**
   Prevents contamination of linen.

6. **Adjust bed to a safe working level, usually waist high. Lower head of bed. Lock bed wheels.**
   When bed is flat, resident can be moved without working against gravity. Adjusting bed level and locking wheels prevents injury to you and resident.

7. **Put on gloves.**
   Prevents you from coming into contact with body fluids.

8. **Loosen top linen from the end of the bed on working side. Unfold bath blanket over the top sheet. Remove top sheet.**

9. **You will make the bed one side at a time. Raise side rail on far side of bed. After raising side rail, go to other side. Help resident to turn onto side, moving away from you toward raised side rail (Fig. 6-43).**

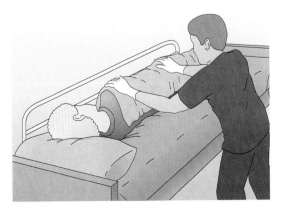

Fig. 6-43.

10. **Loosen bottom soiled linen on working side.**

6

Basic Nursing Skills

6

Basic Nursing Skills

11. **Roll bottom soiled linen toward resident. Tuck it snugly against resident's back.**

    Rolling puts dirtiest surface of linen inward, lessening contamination. The closer the linen is rolled to resident, the easier it is to remove from the other side.

12. **Place and tuck in clean bottom linen. Finish with bottom sheet free of wrinkles. Make hospital corners to keep bottom sheet wrinkle-free (Fig. 6-44).**

    Hospital corners prevent a resident's feet from being restricted by or tangled in linen when getting in and out of bed.

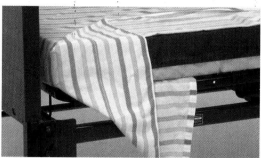

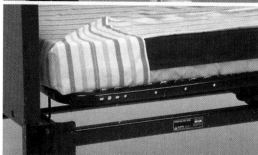

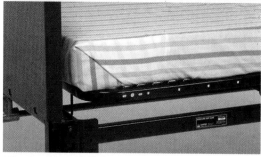

Fig. 6-44. Hospital corners help keep the sheet smooth under the resident.

13. **Smooth the bottom sheet out toward the resident. Be sure there are no wrinkles in the mattress pad. Roll the extra material toward the resident. Tuck it under the resident's body (Fig. 6-45).**

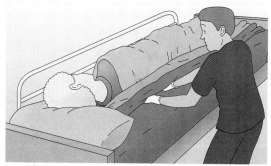

Fig. 6-45.

14. **If using a waterproof pad, unfold it and center it on the bed. Tuck the side near you under the mattress. Smooth it out toward the resident. Tuck as you did with the sheet.**

15. **If using a draw sheet, place it on the bed. Tuck in on your side, smooth, and tuck as you did with the other bedding.**

16. **Raise side rail nearest you. Go to the other side of the bed. Lower side rail. Help resident to turn onto clean bottom sheet (Fig. 6-46).**

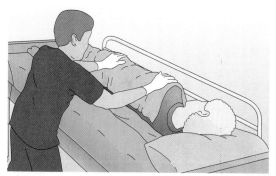

Fig. 6-46.

17. **Loosen soiled linen. Look for personal items. Roll linen from head to foot of bed. Avoid contact with your skin or clothes. Place it in a hamper/bag, at foot of the bed, or in a chair.**

    Always work from cleanest (head of bed) to dirtiest (foot of bed) area to prevent spread of infection. Rolling puts dirtiest surface of linen inward, lessening contamination.

18. **Pull and tuck in clean bottom linen, just like the other side. Finish with bottom sheet free of wrinkles.**

19. Place resident on his back. Keep resident covered and comfortable, with a pillow under the head. Raise side rail.

20. Unfold the top sheet. Place it over the resident. Ask the resident to hold the top sheet. Slip the bath blanket out from underneath. Put it in the hamper/bag.

21. Place a blanket over the top sheet. Tuck the bottom edges of top sheet and blanket under the bottom of the mattress. Make hospital corners on each side. Loosen the top linens over the resident's feet. At the top of the bed, fold the top sheet over the blanket about six inches.

    Loosening the top linens over the feet prevents pressure on the feet, which can cause pressure sores.

22. Remove pillow. Do not hold it near your face. Remove the soiled pillowcase by turning it inside out. Place it in the hamper/bag.

23. With one hand, grasp the clean pillowcase at the closed end. Turn it inside out over your arm. Next, using the same hand that has the pillowcase over it, grasp one narrow edge of the pillow. Pull the pillowcase over it with your free hand (Fig. 6-47). Do the same for any other pillows. Place them under resident's head with open end away from door.

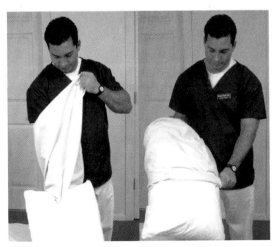

Fig. 6-47.

24. Make resident comfortable.

25. Return bed to appropriate position. Remove privacy measures.

    Lowering the bed provides for safety.

26. Dispose of soiled linen in the proper container.

27. Put call light within resident's reach.

    Allows resident to communicate with staff as necessary.

28. Remove gloves.

29. Wash hands.

    Provides for infection control.

30. Report any changes in resident to the nurse.

    Provides nurse with information to assess resident.

31. Document procedure using facility guidelines.

    What you write is a legal record of what you did. If you don't document it, legally it didn't happen.

Making an unoccupied bed

Equipment: clean linen: mattress pad, fitted or flat bottom sheet, waterproof bed protector if needed, blanket(s), cotton draw sheet, flat top sheet, pillowcase(s), gloves

1. Wash hands.

   Provides for infection control.

2. Place clean linen on clean surface within reach (e.g., bedside stand, overbed table, or chair).

   Prevents contamination of linen.

3. Adjust bed to a safe working level, usually waist high. Put bed in flattest position.

   Allows you to make a neat, wrinkle-free bed.

4. Put on gloves.

   Prevents you from coming into contact with body fluids.

5. Loosen soiled linen. Roll soiled linen (soiled side inside) from head to foot of bed. Avoid contact with your skin or clothes. Place it in a hamper/bag, at foot of the bed, or in chair.

6

Basic Nursing Skills

Always work from cleanest (head of bed) to dirtiest (foot of bed) area to prevent spread of infection. Rolling puts dirtiest surface of linen inward, lessening risk of contamination.

6. **Remove and dispose of gloves. Wash your hands.**

7. **Remake the bed. Spread mattress pad and bottom sheet, tucking under. Make hospital corners to keep bottom sheet wrinkle-free. Put on mattress protector and draw sheet. Smooth, and tuck under sides of bed.**

8. **Place top sheet and blanket over bed. Center these, tuck under end of bed and make hospital corners. Fold down the top sheet over the blanket about six inches. Fold both top sheet and blanket down so resident can easily get into bed. If resident will not be returning to bed immediately, leave bedding up.**

9. **Remove pillows and pillowcases. Put on clean pillowcases (as described above). Replace pillows.**

10. **Return bed to appropriate position.**

11. **Dispose of soiled linen in the proper container.**

12. **Wash your hands.**
    Provides for infection control.

13. **Document procedure using facility guidelines.**
    What you write is a legal record of what you did. If you don't document it, legally it didn't happen.

A **closed bed** is a bed completely made with the bedspread and blankets in place. A closed bed is turned into an **open bed** by folding the linen down to the foot of the bed. Most residents are out of bed much of the day. A closed bed is made until it is time for the resident to go to sleep. Then an open bed is made.

Unit 9. **Explain how to apply non-sterile dressings**

Sterile dressings cover open or draining wounds. A nurse changes these dressings. Non-sterile dressings are applied to dry wounds that have less chance of infection. Nursing assistants may assist with non-sterile dressing changes.

Changing a dry dressing using non-sterile technique

Equipment: package of square gauze dressings, adhesive tape, scissors, 2 pairs of gloves

1. **Wash hands.**
   Provides for infection control.

2. **Identify yourself by name. Identify the resident by name.**
   Resident has right to know identity of his or her caregiver. Addressing resident by name shows respect and establishes correct identification.

3. **Explain procedure to resident. Speak clearly, slowly, and directly. Maintain face-to-face contact whenever possible.**
   Promotes understanding and independence.

4. **Provide for resident's privacy with curtain, screen, or door.**
   Maintains resident's right to privacy and dignity.

5. **Cut pieces of tape long enough to secure the dressing. Hang tape on the edge of a table within reach. Open four-inch gauze square package without touching gauze. Place the opened package on a flat surface.**

6. **Put on gloves.**
   Protects you from coming into contact with body fluids.

7. **Remove soiled dressing by gently peeling tape toward the wound. Lift dressing off the wound. Do not drag it over wound. Observe dressing for any odor. Notice color of the wound. Dispose of**

used dressing in proper container. **Remove and dispose of gloves.**

Avoids disturbing wound healing. Reduces risk of contamination.

8. **Wash hands.**

    Provides for infection control.

9. **Put on new gloves. Touching only outer edges of new four-inch gauze, remove it from package. Apply it to wound. Tape gauze in place. Secure firmly (Fig. 6-48).**

    Keeps gauze as clean as possible.

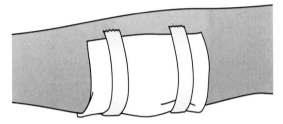

Fig. 6-48.

10. **Remove and dispose of gloves properly.**

11. **Remove privacy measures.**

12. **Before leaving, place call light within resident's reach.**

    Allows resident to communicate with staff as necessary.

13. **Wash hands.**

    Provides for infection control.

14. **Report any changes in resident to the nurse.**

    Provides nurse with information to assess resident.

15. **Document procedure according to facility guidelines.**

    What you write is a legal record of what you did. If you don't document it, legally it didn't happen.

seven

Nutrition and Hydration

Unit 1. **Identify the six basic nutrients and explain MyPyramid**

Good nutrition is very important. **Nutrition** is how the body uses food to maintain health. Bodies need a well-balanced diet with nutrients and plenty of fluids. This helps us grow new cells, maintain normal body function, and have energy. Good nutrition in early life helps ensure good health later. For the ill or elderly, a well-balanced diet helps maintain muscle and skin tissues and prevent pressure sores. A good diet also promotes healing. It helps us cope with stress.

The Six Basic Nutrients

The body needs the following nutrients for growth and development:

1. **Protein**. Proteins are part of every body cell. They are essential for tissue growth and repair. Proteins are also an alternate supply of energy for the body.

Sources include fish, seafood, poultry, meat, eggs, milk, cheese, nuts, peas, and dried beans or legumes (Fig. 7-1).

Whole grain cereals, pastas, rice, and breads contain some proteins of lower quality. These must be complemented by a small quantity of the more complete proteins. Beans and rice or cereal and milk are examples of complementary proteins.

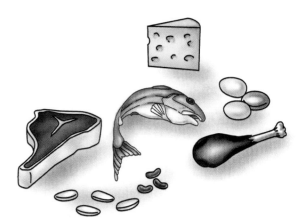

Fig. 7-1. **Sources of protein.**

2. **Carbohydrates**. Carbohydrates supply the fuel for the body's energy needs. They help the body use fat efficiently. Carbohydrates also provide fiber, which is necessary for bowel elimination.

Carbohydrates can be divided into two basic types: complex and simple carbohydrates. Complex carbohydrates are found in foods such as bread, cereal, potatoes, rice, pasta, vegetables, and fruits. Simple carbohydrates are found in foods such as sugars, sweets, syrups, and jellies. Simple carbohydrates do not have the same nutritional value as complex carbohydrates do (Fig. 7-2).

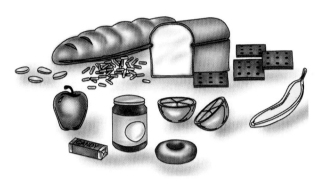

Fig. 7-2. Sources of carbohydrates.

The only value of simple carbohydrates is as energy for people who eat very little or are malnourished. In others, simple carbohydrates are stored as fat.

3. **Fats.** Fat helps the body store energy. Body fat also provides insulation. It protects body organs. Fats help the body absorb vitamins. Fats also add flavor to food. Excess fat in the diet is stored as fat in the body.

Examples of fats are butter, margarine, salad dressings, oils, and animal fats in meats, fowl, and fish (Fig. 7-3).

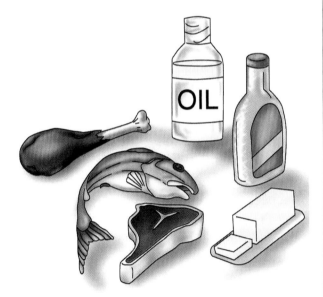

Fig. 7-3. Sources of fat.

Monounsaturated vegetable fats (including olive oil and canola oil) and polyunsaturated vegetable fats (including corn and safflower oils) are healthier kinds of fats. Saturated fats, including animal fats like butter, bacon and other fatty meats, are not as healthy. They should be limited.

♥ *Saturated fats raise the level of blood cholesterol. This can contribute to circulatory disorders.*

4. **Vitamins.** Vitamins are substances the body needs to function. The body cannot produce most vitamins. They can only be obtained from food, and are essential to body functions. Vitamins A, D, E, and K are fat-soluble vitamins. This means they are carried and stored in body fat. Vitamins B and C are water-soluble vitamins. They are broken down by water in our bodies. They cannot be stored in the body. They are eliminated in urine and feces.

5. **Minerals.** Minerals form and maintain cells. They provide energy and control processes. Zinc, iron, calcium, and magnesium are some minerals. Minerals are found in many foods.

6. **Water.** One-half to two-thirds of our body weight is water. We need about eight glasses, or 64 ounces, of water or other fluids a day. Water is the most essential nutrient for life. Without it, a person can only live a few days. Water assists in the digestion and absorption of food. It helps with waste elimination. Through perspiration, water helps maintain normal body temperature. Keeping enough fluid in our bodies is necessary for good health.

Most foods have several nutrients. No one food has all the nutrients needed for a healthy body. This is why it is important to eat a daily diet that is well-balanced. There is not one single dietary plan that is right for everyone. People have different nutritional needs depending upon their age, gender, and activity level.

7

Nutrition and Hydration

In 1980, the U.S. Department of Agriculture (USDA) developed the Food Guide Pyramid to help promote healthy eating practices. In 2005, in response to new scientific information about nutrition and health and new technology for support tools, MyPyramid was developed (Fig. 7-4). MyPyramid replaces the Food Guide Pyramid. MyPyramid is a personalized version of the Food Guide Pyramid that offers individual plans based on age, gender, and activity level.

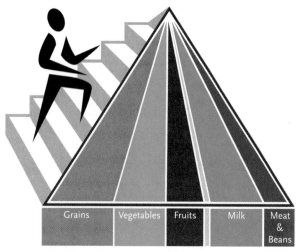

Fig. 7-4. MyPyramid was developed to help promote healthy eating practices. It offers individual plans based on age, gender and activity level.

The Pyramid is made up of six bands of different widths and colors. Each color represents a food group—orange for grains, green for vegetables, maroon for fruits, yellow for oils, blue for milk, and purple for meat and beans. The different widths indicate that not all groups should make up an equal part of a healthy diet. The orange band, grains, is the widest. This means that grains should make up the highest proportion of the diet. The smaller bands, such as the purple band representing meat and beans, should make up a smaller part of foods eaten. The smallest band, the yellow one, represents oils. Oils contain essential fatty acids. However, this band is not emphasized because the body needs fats and oils in smaller quantities.

The bands of the Pyramid are wide at the bottom and narrow into a point at the top. This is a reminder that there are a great variety of foods that make up each group. Many choices are available to help meet the daily requirements. Foods that are nutrient-dense and low in fat and calories should form the "base" of a healthy diet. They are represented by the wide base of the Pyramid. Foods that are high in fat and sugar and have less nutritional value are at the narrow top. They should be eaten less often.

The new Pyramid also emphasizes the importance of physical activity, as represented by the figure climbing the stairs. Physical activity goes hand-in-hand with diet to make up an overall healthy lifestyle. The USDA recommends at least 30 minutes per day of vigorous activity for everyone. Sixty minutes or more is even better.

Grains. The grains group includes all foods made from wheat, rice, oats, cornmeal, and barley. Examples are bread, pasta, oatmeal, breakfast cereals, tortillas, and grits. One slice of bread, one cup of ready-to-eat cereal, or ½ cup of cooked rice, pasta, or cooked cereal can be considered a one-ounce equivalent from the grains group.

There are two subgroups of grains: whole grains and refined grains. Whole grains contain the entire grain kernel. Refined grains have been milled. This is a process that removes the bran and germ. This gives grain a finer texture and improves its shelf life but also removes dietary fiber, iron, and many B vitamins. At least half of all grains consumed should be whole grains. Words on food labels that ensure that grains are whole grains are: brown rice, wild rice, bulgur, oatmeal, whole-grain corn, whole oats, whole wheat, and whole rye.

Vegetables. The vegetable group includes all fresh, frozen, canned and dried vegetables and vegetable juices. One cup of raw or cooked vegetables or vegetable juice or two cups of raw leafy greens can be considered as one cup from the vegetable group. There are five subgroups within the vegetable group. They are organized by nutritional content. These are dark green vegetables, orange vegetables, dry beans and peas, starchy vegetables, and other vegetables. A variety of vegetables from these subgroups should be eaten every day. Dark green vegetables, orange vegetables, and dried beans and peas have the best nutritional content.

Vegetables are low in fat and calories and have no cholesterol (although sauces and seasonings may add fat, calories and cholesterol). They are good sources of dietary fiber, potassium, Vitamin A, Vitamin E, and Vitamin C.

Fruits. The fruit group includes all fresh, frozen, canned and dried fruits and fruit juices. One cup of fruit or 100% fruit juice or ½ cup of dried fruit can be considered as one cup from the fruit group. Most choices should be whole or cut-up fruit rather than juice for the additional dietary fiber provided.

Fruits, like vegetables, are naturally low in fat, sodium and calories and have no cholesterol. They are important sources of dietary fiber and many nutrients, including folic acid and Vitamin C.

Milk. The milk group includes all fluid milk products and foods made from milk that retain their calcium content, such as yogurt and cheese (Fig. 7-5). Foods made from milk that have little to no calcium, such as cream cheese, cream, and butter, are not part of the group. Most milk group choices should be

fat-free or low-fat. One cup of milk or yogurt, one-and-a-half ounces of natural cheese, or two ounces of processed cheese can be considered as one cup from the milk group.

Foods in the milk group provide nutrients that are vital for the health and maintenance of your body. These nutrients include calcium, potassium, Vitamin D, and protein. Calcium is used for building bones and teeth and in maintaining bone mass. Milk products are the primary source of calcium in American diets.

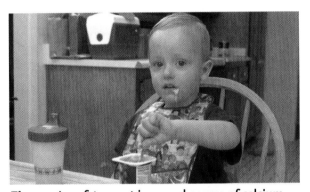

Fig. 7-5. Low-fat yogurt is a good source of calcium.

Meat and Beans. One ounce of lean meat, poultry, or fish, one egg, one tablespoon peanut butter, ¼ cup cooked dry beans, or ½ ounce of nuts or seeds can be considered as one ounce equivalent from the meat and beans group. Dry beans and peas can be included as part of this group or part of the vegetable group. If meat is eaten regularly, dry beans and peas should be included with vegetables. If not, they should be included as part of this group.

Most meat and poultry choices should be lean or low-fat. Diets that are high in saturated fats raise "bad" cholesterol levels in the blood. Some food choices in this group are high in saturated fat. These include fatty cuts of beef, pork, and lamb; regular (75% to 85% lean) ground beef; regular sausages, hot dogs, and bacon; some luncheon meats such as regular bologna and salami; and some poultry such as duck. These foods should be limited to help keep blood cholesterol levels healthy.

Fish, nuts, and seeds contain healthy oils. These foods are a good choice instead of meat or poultry. Some nuts and seeds (flax, walnuts) are excellent sources of essential fatty acids. These acids may reduce the risk of cardiovascular disease. Some (sunflower seeds, almonds, hazelnuts) are good sources of Vitamin E.

Oils. Oils include fats from many different plants and from fish that are liquid at room temperature, such as canola, corn, olive, soybean and sunflower oil. Some foods are naturally high in oils, like nuts, olives, some fish, and avocados. Foods that are mainly oil include mayonnaise, certain salad dressings, and soft margarine.

Most of the fats you eat should be polyunsaturated (PUFA) or monounsaturated (MUFA) fats. Oils are the major source of MUFAs and PUFAs in the diet. PUFAs contain some fatty acids that are necessary for health. These are called "essential fatty acids."

Most Americans consume enough oil in the foods they eat, such as nuts, fish, cooking oil, and salad dressings.

Activity. Physical activity and nutrition work together for better health. Being active increases the amount of calories burned. As people age, their metabolism slows. Maintaining energy balance requires moving more and eating less. For health benefits, physical activity should be moderate or vigorous and add up to at least 30 minutes a day.

For more information on MyPyramid, visit www.mypyramid.gov.

Unit 2. **Demonstrate an awareness of regional, cultural, and religious food preferences**

Culture, ethnicity, income, education, religion, and geography all affect attitudes about nutrition. Food preferences may be formed by what you ate as a child, by what tastes good, or by personal beliefs about what should be eaten (Fig. 7-6). Some people choose not to eat any animals or animal products, such as steak, chicken, butter, or eggs. These people are vegetarians or vegans.

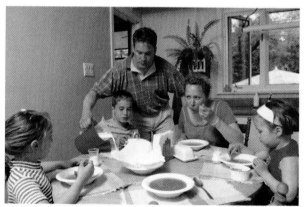

Fig. 7-6. Food likes and dislikes are influenced by what you ate as a child.

RA *Residents' Rights include the right to make choices. This means that you must honor a resident's personal beliefs about selecting and avoiding specific foods.*

The region or culture you grow up in often affects your food preference. People from the southwestern U.S. may like spicy food. "Southern cooking" may include fried foods, like fried chicken or fried okra. Religious beliefs affect diet, too. Some Muslim and Jewish people do not eat any pork. Some Mormons may not drink alcohol, coffee, or tea.

Whatever your residents' food preferences may be, respect them. Never make fun of a personal preference. If you notice that certain food is not being eaten—no matter how small—report it to the nurse.

Unit 3. Explain special diets

A doctor sometimes places residents who are ill on special diets. These diets are known as **therapeutic**, **modified**, or **special diets**. After a doctor prescribes a special diet, the dietitian plans the diet. Doctors may order supplementary diets for residents who do not eat enough. Diets are also used for weight control and food allergies.

The dietary department makes diet cards (Fig. 7-7). **Diet cards** list the resident's name and information about special diets, allergies, likes and dislikes and any other instructions.

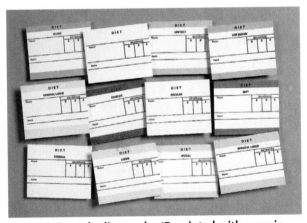

Fig. 7-7. Sample diet cards. (Reprinted with permission of Briggs Corporation, Des Moines, IA, 800-247-2343.)

Examples of special diets are listed below:

Low-Sodium Diet. Residents with heart disease, kidney disease, or fluid retention may be placed on a low-sodium diet. Many foods have sodium, but people are most familiar with it as an ingredient in table salt. Salt is the first food to be restricted in a low-sodium diet because it is high in sodium.

For residents on a low-sodium diet, salt will not be used. Salt shakers or packets will not be on the diet tray. Common abbreviations for this diet found on diet cards are "Low Na," which means low sodium, or "NAS," which stands for "No Added Salt."

Fluid-Restricted Diets. The fluid taken into the body through food and fluids must equal the fluid that leaves the body through perspiration, stool, urine, and expiration. This is **fluid balance**. When fluid intake is greater than fluid output, body tissue becomes swollen with excess fluid. People with severe heart disease or kidney disease may have difficulty processing fluid. To prevent further damage, doctors may restrict fluid intake. For residents on fluid restriction, you will need to measure and document exact amounts of fluid intake and report excesses to the nurse.

Do not offer additional fluids or foods that count as fluids, such as ice cream, puddings, gelatin, etc. If the resident complains of thirst or requests fluids, tell the nurse. The abbreviation for this diet is "RF." This stands for "Restrict Fluids."

Low-Protein Diet. People who have kidney disease may be on low-protein diets. Protein is restricted because it breaks down into compounds that may further damage the kidneys. The extent of the restrictions depends on the stage of the disease and if the resident is on dialysis.

Low-Fat/Low-Cholesterol Diet. People who have high levels of cholesterol in their blood are at risk for heart attacks and heart disease. People with gallbladder disease, diseases that interfere with fat digestion, and liver disease are also placed on low-fat/low-cholesterol diets. Low-fat/low-cholesterol diets permit skim milk, low-fat cottage cheese, fish, white meat of turkey and chicken, veal, and vegetable fats (especially monounsaturated fats such as olive, canola, and peanut oils) (Fig. 7-8).

People who have gallbladder disease or other digestive problems may be placed on a diet that restricts all fats. A common abbreviation for this diet is "Low-Fat/Low-Chol."

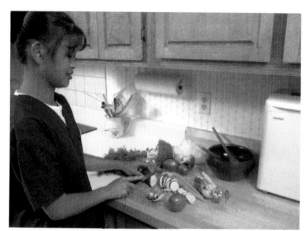

Fig. 7-8. Vegetables are an important part of a low-fat/low-cholesterol diet.

Modified Calorie Diet for Weight Management. Some residents may need to reduce calories to lose weight or prevent additional weight gain. Other residents may need to increase calories because of malnutrition, surgery, illness, or fever. Common abbreviations for this diet are "Low-Cal" or "High-Cal."

Dietary Management of Diabetes. Calories and carbohydrates are carefully controlled in the diets of diabetic residents (see chapter 8 for more information on this disorder). Protein and fats are also regulated. The types of foods and the amounts are determined by nutritional and energy needs.

A dietitian and the resident will make up a meal plan. It will include all the right types and amounts of food for each day. The resident uses exchange lists, or lists of similar foods that can substitute for one another, to make up a menu. Using meal plans and exchange lists, a person with diabetes can control his diet while still making food choices.

To keep their blood glucose levels near normal, diabetic residents must eat the right amount of the right type of food at the right time. They must eat all that is served. Encourage them to do so. Do not offer other foods without the nurse's approval. If a resident will not eat what is directed, or if you think that he or she is not following the diet, tell the nurse.

A diabetic's meal tray may have artificial sweetener, low-calorie jelly, and maple syrup When serving coffee or tea to a diabetic resident, use artificial sweeteners rather than sugar. The common abbreviations for this diet on a diet card are "NCS," which stands for "No Concentrated Sweets," or the amount of calories followed by the abbreviation "ADA," which stands for American Diabetic Association.

Diets may also be modified in consistency.

Liquid Diet. A liquid diet consists of foods that are in a liquid state at body temperature. Liquid diets are usually ordered as "clear" or "full." A clear liquid diet includes clear juices, broth, gelatin, and popsicles. A full liquid diet includes all the liquids served on a clear liquid diet with the addition of cream soups, milk, and ice cream. A liquid diet is usually ordered for a short time due to a medical condition or before or after a test or surgery.

Soft Diet. The soft diet is soft in texture and consists of soft or chopped foods that are easy to chew and swallow. Doctors order this diet for residents who have trouble chewing and swallowing due to dental problems or other medical conditions.

Pureed Diet. To **puree** a food means to chop, blend, or grind it into a thick paste of baby food consistency. The food should be thick enough to hold its form in the mouth. This diet does not require a person to chew his or her food. A pureed diet is often used for people who have trouble chewing and/or swallowing more textured foods.

The abbreviation "NPO" stands for "Nothing by Mouth." This means that a resident is not allowed to have anything to eat or drink. Some residents have such a severe problem with swallowing that it is unsafe to give them anything by mouth. These types of residents will receive nutrition through a feeding tube or intravenously. See unit 9 for more information on swallowing problems.

Some residents may be NPO for a short time before a medical test or surgery. You need to know this abbreviation. Never offer any food or drink to a resident with this order.

Unit 4. Understand the importance of observing and reporting a resident's diet

It is very important to identify the resident before serving a meal tray or helping with feeding. Feeding a resident the wrong food can cause serious problems, even death. Before you deliver trays or plates, check them closely. Make sure that you have the correct resident and the correct food and beverages for that person. Trays and plates should also be closely checked for added sugar and salt packets (Fig. 7-9). Always check trays for dentures, glasses, and hearing aids before removing them.

Be aware of residents who are diabetic or have heart conditions. They will be on special diets. Their families may not know or understand about food restrictions. Families often bring treats into the facility for their loved ones. Watch for foods in residents' rooms that are not permitted by their doctors. Report any problems to the nurse.

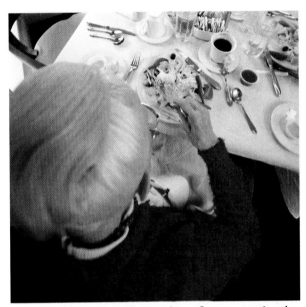

Fig. 7-9. **Observe residents' plates for any restricted food.**

Food trays and plates should also be observed after the meal. It is important to observe what and how much the resident is eating. This helps identify residents with poor appetites. It may also signal illness, a problem, such as dentures that do not fit properly, or a change in food preferences.

All facilities keep track of how much food and liquid a resident consumes. The method varies. Some facilities use a percentage method. Below is one example of a percentage method:

- "R" Refused = 0% No food is eaten
- "P" Poor = 25% Very little food is eaten
- "F" Fair = 50% Half of the food is eaten
- "G" Good = 75% Most of the food is eaten
- "A" All = 100% Entire meal is eaten

Other facilities may document the percentage of specific foods eaten—protein, carbohydrates, fats, etc. Follow your facility's policy. Document food intake very carefully. Accuracy is important.

Unit 5. Describe how to assist residents in maintaining fluid balance

Most residents should be encouraged to drink at least eight glasses, or 64 ounces, of water or other fluids a day. Water is essential for life (Fig. 7-10). The sense of thirst can lessen as people age. Remind your elderly residents to drink fluids often. Some residents will drink more fluids if they are offered them in smaller amounts, rather than in one large glassful. Residents may have an order to force fluids (FF) or restrict fluids (RF) because of medical conditions. **Force fluids** means to encourage the resident to drink more fluids. **Restrict fluids** means the person is allowed to drink, but must limit the daily amount to a level set by the doctor. Make sure you know which residents have these special orders.

Dehydration occurs when a person does not have enough fluid in the body. Dehydration is a major problem among the elderly, in and out of nursing homes. People can become dehydrated if they do not drink enough or if they have diarrhea or are vomiting. Preventing dehydration is important.

Observing and Reporting Dehydration

Report any of these immediately:

- resident drinks less than six 8 oz. glasses of liquid per day

- resident drinks little or no fluids at meals

- resident needs help drinking from a cup or glass

- resident has trouble swallowing liquids

- resident has frequent vomiting, diarrhea, or fever

- resident is easily confused or tired

Report any of these symptoms:

- dry mouth

- cracked lips

- sunken eyes

- dark urine

- strong-smelling urine

- weight loss

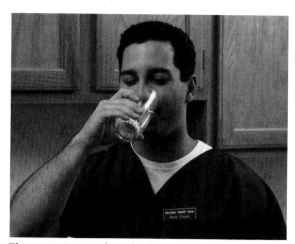

Fig. 7-10. Remember, drinking plenty of water is good for you, too!

Guidelines
Preventing Dehydration

- Report observations and warning signs to the nurse immediately.

- Encourage residents to drink every time you see them (Fig. 7-11).

- Offer fresh water or other fluids often. Offer drinks that the resident enjoys. Honor personal preferences.

- Record fluid intake and output.

- Ice chips, frozen flavored ice sticks, and gelatin are also liquids. Offer them often. Do not offer ice chips or sticks if a resident has a swallowing problem.

- If appropriate, offer sips of liquid between bites of food at meals and snacks.

- Make sure pitcher and cup are near enough and light enough for the resident to lift.

- Offer assistance if resident cannot drink without help. Use adaptive cups as needed.

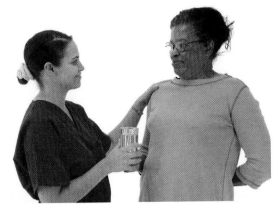

Fig. 7-11. Encouraging residents to drink every time you see them can help prevent dehydration.

Serving fresh water

Equipment: water pitcher, ice scoop, glass, straw, gloves

1. **Wash hands.**

   Provides for infection control.

2. **Identify yourself by name. Identify the resident by name.**

   Resident has right to know identity of his or her caregiver. Addressing resident by name shows respect and establishes correct identification.

3. **Put on gloves.**

   Promotes infection control.

4. **Scoop ice into water pitcher. Add fresh water.**

5. **Use and store ice scoop properly:**

   Do not allow ice to touch hand and fall back into container.

   Place scoop in proper receptacle after each use.

   Avoids contamination of ice.

6. **Take pitcher to resident.**

7. **Pour glass of water for resident. Leave pitcher and glass at the bedside.**

   Encourages resident to maintain hydration.

8. **Make sure that pitcher and glass are light enough for resident to lift. Leave a straw if the resident desires.**

   Demonstrates understanding of resident's abilities and/or limitations. Prevents dehydration.

9. **Before leaving resident, place call light within resident's reach.**

   Allows resident to communicate with staff as necessary.

10. **Remove gloves.**

11. **Wash hands.**

    Provides for infection control.

👁 *You must be very careful not to contaminate the ice each time you scoop it. Never touch the ice and allow it to fall back into the container. Make sure the scoop is placed in the proper place after each use.*

Fluid overload occurs when the body cannot handle the fluid consumed. This often affects people with heart or kidney disease.

Observing and Reporting Fluid Overload

- swelling/edema of extremities (ankles, feet, fingers, hands); **edema** is swelling caused by excess fluid in body tissues

- weight gain (daily weight gain of one to two pounds)

- less urine output

- shortness of breath

- increased heart rate

- skin that appears tight, smooth, and shiny

Unit 6. List ways to identify and prevent unintended weight loss

Just like dehydration, unintended weight loss is a serious problem for the elderly. Weight loss can mean that the resident has a serious medical condition. It can lead to skin breakdown. This leads to pressure sores. It is very important to report any weight loss you notice, no matter how small. If a resident has diabetes, chronic obstructive pulmonary disease, cancer, HIV, or other diseases, he is at a greater risk for malnutrition. (See chapter 8 for more information.)

Observing and Reporting Unintended Weight Loss:

Report any of these immediately:

- resident needs help eating or drinking
- resident eats less than 70% of meals/snacks
- resident has mouth pain
- resident has dentures that do not fit
- resident has difficulty chewing or swallowing
- resident coughs or chokes while eating
- resident is sad, has crying spells, or withdraws from others
- resident is confused, wanders, or paces

Guidelines
Preventing Unintended Weight Loss

- Report observations and warning signs to the nurse.
- Encourage residents to eat. Talk about food being served in a positive tone of voice and with positive words.
- Honor residents' food likes and dislikes.
- Offer different kinds of foods and beverages.
- Help residents who have trouble feeding themselves.
- Food should look, taste, and smell good. The person may have a poor sense of taste and smell.
- Season foods to residents' preferences.
- Allow time for residents to finish eating.
- Tell the nurse if residents have trouble using utensils.

- Record meal/snack intake.
- Give oral care before and after meals.
- Position residents sitting upright for feeding.
- If resident has had a loss of appetite and/or seems sad, ask about it.

Regulations require that the intake of food and fluids be monitored to prevent malnutrition and dehydration. Nursing assistants must assist residents with eating and drinking so that they are nourished and hydrated.

Unit 7. Identify ways to promote appetites at mealtime

Mealtime is an important part of a resident's day. This is especially true because weight loss and malnutrition issues are common among the elderly. Illness, pain, and medications may cause loss of appetite.

Not only is mealtime the time for getting proper nourishment, but it is also a time for socializing. Weight loss and dehydration are not the only problems residents have. Loneliness and boredom cause other kinds of suffering. You can help the whole person.

Encourage healthy eating. Do all that you can to promote a resident's appetite. Mealtime should be pleasant (Fig. 7-12). Use these tips to help promote appetites and to make dining enjoyable:

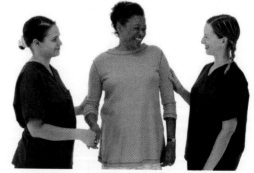

Fig. 7-12. Nursing assistants play an important part in making mealtime enjoyable for residents.

Guidelines
Promoting Appetites

- Check the environment. Address any odors. The temperature should be comfortable. Keep noise level low.

- Encourage the use of dentures, glasses, and hearing aids. If these are damaged, notify the nurse.

- Offer a trip to the bathroom or help with toileting before eating.

- Help residents wash hands before eating.

- Give oral care before eating.

- Properly position residents for eating. Usually, the proper position is upright, at a 90-degree angle. If residents use a wheelchair, make sure they are sitting at a table that is the right height. Most facilities have adjustable tables for wheelchairs.

- If a resident has poor sitting balance, seat him or her in a regular dining room chair with armrests, rather than in a wheelchair. Proper position in chair means hips at a 90-degree angle, knees flexed, and feet and arms fully supported. Push chair under the table. Place forearms on the table. If a resident tends to lean to one side, ask him or her to keep elbows on the table.

- If a resident has poor neck control, a neck brace may be used to stabilize the head. Use assistive devices as needed.

- Seat residents next to their friends or people with like interests. Encourage conversation.

- Serve food at the correct temperature.

- Plates and trays should look appetizing.

- Give the resident proper eating tools. Use adaptive utensils if needed. (See chapter 9.)

- Be cheerful, positive, and helpful. Make conversation if the resident wishes (Fig. 7-13).

- Give more food when requested.

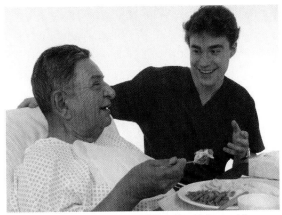

Fig. 7-13. **Be pleasant and friendly while residents are eating.**

Unit 8. Demonstrate ways to feed residents

One duty you will have is helping residents with their meals. Residents will need different levels of help. Some residents will not need any help. Some residents will only need help setting up. They may need help opening cartons and cutting and seasoning their food. Once that is done, they can feed themselves. Check in with these residents from time to time to see if they need anything else.

Some residents will need some help. Residents who have had a stroke, who have Parkinson's disease, Alzheimer's disease or other dementias, who have had head trauma, or who are confused or blind may benefit from physical and verbal cues. You will learn more about these diseases in chapter 8. The hand-over-hand approach is an example of physical cuing. If a resident can help lift the utensils, put your hand over his to help with eating. After the spoon is in the resident's hand, place your hand over the resident's hand. Help the resident in getting some food on the spoon. Steer the spoon from the food to the mouth and back. This promotes independence.

Other residents will be completely unable to feed themselves. It will be your job to feed them. Residents who must be fed are often embarrassed and depressed about their dependence on another person. Be sensitive to this. Give residents privacy while they are eating. Do not rush them. Always encourage residents to do whatever they can for themselves. For example, if a resident can hold and use a napkin, she should. If she can hold and eat finger foods, offer them. There are devices that can help residents eat (Fig. 7-14). Cups with lids to avoid spills and utensils with thick handles that are easier to hold are two examples. More adaptive devices are shown in chapter 9.

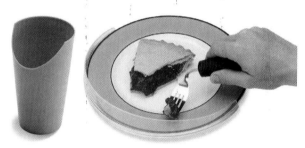

Fig. 7-14. Sample assistive devices for eating. (Photos courtesy of North Coast Medical, Inc., 800-821-9319, www.ncmedical.com.)

RA *If a resident does not want to use a clothing protector while eating, that is his or her right. Respect the resident's wishes.*

Guidelines
Assisting a Resident with Eating

- Never treat the resident like a child. This is embarrassing and disrespectful. It is hard for many people to accept help with feeding. Be supportive and encouraging.

- Sit at a resident's eye level. Make eye contact with the resident.

- If the resident wishes, allow time for prayer.

- Verify that you have the right resident. Check the diet card against the resident's ID bracelet or whatever method is used by the facility to identify residents. Also, check that the diet on the tray is correct.

- Do not touch food to test its temperature. Put your hand over the dish to sense the heat of food. If you think the food is too hot, do not blow on it to cool it. Offer other food to give it time to cool. Remove dishes from metal hot plates.

- Cut foods and pour liquids as needed.

- Identify the foods and fluids that are in front of the resident. Call pureed foods by the correct name. For example, ask, "Would you like some green beans?" rather than referring to it as "some green stuff."

- Ask the resident what he wants to eat first. Allow him to make the choice, even if he wants to eat dessert first.

- Do not mix foods unless the resident prefers it.

- Do not rush the meal. Allow time for the resident to chew and swallow each bite. Be relaxed.

- Make conversation. Use appropriate topics, such as the news, weather, the resident's life, things the resident enjoys, and food preferences. Say positive things about the food being served, such as, "This smells really good," and, "The [type of food] looks so fresh."

- Give the resident your full attention.

- Alternate food and drink. Alternating cold and hot foods or bland foods and sweets can help increase appetite.

RA *Residents have the right to refuse food and drink. Residents also have the right to ask for and receive different food. If the resident wants a different food from what is being served, honor this request. Tell the dietitian so that an alternative may be offered.*

Feeding a resident who cannot feed self

Equipment: meal tray, clothing protector, 1-2 washcloths

1. **Wash hands.**
   Provides for infection control.

2. **Identify yourself by name. Identify the resident by name.**
Resident has right to know identity of his or her caregiver. Addressing resident by name shows respect and establishes correct identification.

3. **Explain procedure to resident. Speak clearly, slowly, and directly. Maintain face-to-face contact whenever possible.**
Promotes understanding and independence.

4. **Pick up diet card. Verify that resident has received the right tray.**
Tray should only contain foods, fluids, and condiments permitted on the diet.

5. **Help resident to wash hands if resident cannot do it on her own.**
Promotes good hygiene and infection control.

6. **Adjust bed height to where you will be to able to sit at resident's eye level. Lock bed wheels.**

7. **Raise the head of the bed. Make sure resident is in an upright sitting position (at a 90-degree angle).**
Promotes ease of swallowing. Prevents aspiration of food and beverage.

8. **Help resident to put on clothing protector, if desired.**
Protects resident's clothing from food and beverage spills.

9. **Sit facing resident. Sit at resident's eye level (Fig. 7-15). Sit on the stronger side if resident has one-sided weakness.**
Promotes good communication. Lets resident know that he or she will not be rushed while eating.

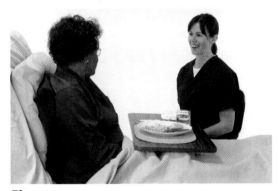

Fig. 7-15.

10. **Offer drink of beverage. Offer different types of food, allowing for resident's preferences. (Do not feed all of one type before offering another type.)**
Resident has right to make decisions.

11. **Offer the food in bite-sized pieces. Report any swallowing problems to the nurse immediately (Fig. 7-16).**
Small pieces are easier to chew and lessens the risk of choking.

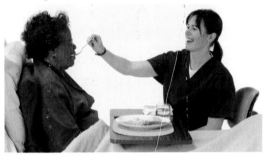

Fig. 7-16.

12. **Make sure resident's mouth is empty before next bite or sip.**
Lessens risk of choking.

13. **Offer beverage to resident throughout the meal.**
Promotes ease of swallowing.

14. **Talk with the resident during the meal (Fig. 7-17).**
Makes mealtime more enjoyable.

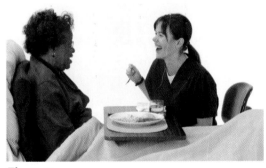

Fig. 7-17.

15. **Use washcloths to wipe food from resident's mouth and hands as needed during the meal. Wipe again at the end of the meal (Fig. 7-18).**
Maintains resident's dignity.

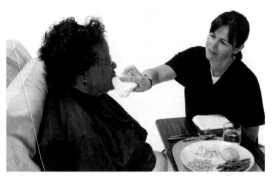

Fig. 7-18.

16. **Remove clothing protector if used. Dispose of in proper container.**

17. **Remove food tray. Check for eyeglasses, dentures, or any personal items before removing tray.**

18. **Make resident comfortable. Make sure sheets are free from wrinkles and the bed free from crumbs.**

    Wrinkles and crumbs can cause skin breakdown.

19. **Return bed to proper position.**

20. **Before leaving, place call light within resident's reach.**

    Allows resident to communicate with staff as necessary.

21. **Wash hands.**

    Provides for infection control.

22. **Report any changes in resident to the nurse.**

    Provides nurse with information to assess resident.

23. **Document procedure using facility guidelines.**

    What you write is a legal record of what you did. If you don't document it, legally it didn't happen.

👁 *You must offer fluid to the resident throughout the meal. Remember to raise the head of the bed to help prevent aspiration.*

Unit 9. Describe eating and swallowing problems a resident may have

Dysphagia means difficulty in swallowing.

You need to be able to recognize and report signs that a resident has a swallowing problem. Signs and symptoms of swallowing problems include:

- coughing during or after meals
- choking during meals
- dribbling saliva, food, or fluid from the mouth
- food residue inside the mouth or cheeks during and after meals
- gurgling sound in voice during or after meals or loss of voice
- slow eating
- avoidance of eating
- spitting out pieces of food
- several swallows needed per mouthful
- frequent throat clearing during and after meals
- watering eyes when eating or drinking
- food or fluid coming up into the nose
- visible effort to swallow
- shorter or more rapid breathing while eating or drinking
- difficulty chewing food
- difficulty swallowing medications

If you notice any signs of swallowing problems, notify the nurse immediately.

Residents may have conditions that make eating or swallowing difficult. A stroke, or CVA, can cause weakness on one side of the body and paralysis. Nerve and muscle damage from head and neck cancer, multiple sclerosis, Parkinson's or Alzheimer's disease may be present. You will learn more about these diseases in chapter 8. If a resident has trouble swallowing, soft foods and thickened liquids will be served. A straw or special cup will help make swallowing easier.

Thickening improves the ability to control fluid in the mouth and throat. Special products are used for thickening. A doctor orders the necessary thickness after the resident has been evaluated by a speech therapist. Some beverages arrive already thickened from the dietary department. In other facilities, the thickening agent is added on the nursing unit before serving. If thickening is ordered, it must be used with all liquids. You need to know what thickened liquids mean. Do not offer these residents regular liquids. Never offer a water pitcher to a resident who must have thickened liquids. Follow the directions for each resident.

Three basic thickened consistencies are:

1. **Nectar Thick**: This consistency is thicker than water. It is the thickness of a thick juice, such as a pear nectar or tomato juice. A resident can drink this from a cup.

2. **Honey Thick**: This consistency has the thickness of honey. It will pour very slowly. A resident usually uses a spoon to consume it.

3. **Pudding Thick**: With this consistency, the liquids have become semi-solid, much like pudding. A spoon should stand up straight in the glass when put into the middle of the drink. A resident must consume these liquids with a spoon.

Swallowing problems put residents at high risk for choking on food or drink. Inhaling food or drink into the lungs is called **aspiration**. Aspiration can cause pneumonia or death. Alert the nurse immediately if any problems occur while feeding.

Guidelines
Preventing Aspiration

- Position residents properly when eating.

They must sit in a straight, upright position. Do not try to feed residents in a reclining position.

- Offer small pieces of food or small spoonfuls of pureed food.

- Feed resident slowly.

- Place food in the non-paralyzed, or unaffected, side of the mouth.

- Make sure mouth is empty before each bite of food or sip of drink.

- Residents should stay in the upright position for about 30 minutes after eating and drinking.

When a person is completely unable to swallow, he or she may be fed through a tube. A **nasogastric tube** is inserted into the nose and goes to the stomach. A tube can also be placed through the skin directly into the stomach. This is called a **PEG** (Percutaneous Endoscopic Gastrostomy) **tube**. The opening in the stomach and abdomen is called a **gastrostomy** (Fig. 7-19). Tube feedings are used when residents cannot swallow but can digest food. Conditions that may prevent swallowing include coma, cancer, stroke, refusal to eat, or extreme weakness.

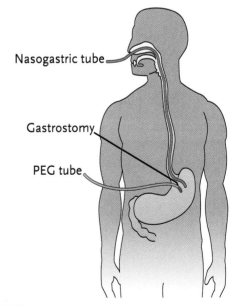

Nasogastric tube

Gastrostomy

PEG tube

Fig. 7-19.

If a person's digestive system does not function properly, **hyperalimentation** or **total parenteral nutrition** (**TPN**) may be needed. With TPN, a resident receives nutrients directly into the bloodstream. It bypasses the digestive system.

NAs never insert tubes, do the feeding, or clean the tubes. You may assemble equipment and supplies and hand them to the nurse. You may position the resident. You may also discard used equipment and supplies, clean, or store equipment and supplies.

Guidelines
Tube Feedings

- Check often to make sure that tubing is not kinked or pulled.

- Check to make sure that the resident is not resting on the tubing.

- The resident may have an order for nothing by mouth, or NPO. Be aware of this.

- The tube is only inserted and removed by a doctor or nurse. If it comes out, report it immediately.

- A doctor will prescribe the type and amount of feeding. Do not place anything else into the tube. The feedings will be in a liquid form. The dietary department prepares them or they are prepackaged.

- During the feeding, the resident should remain in a sitting position with the head of the bed elevated about 45 degrees to help prevent aspiration.

- If your resident must remain in bed for long periods during feedings, provide good skin care to prevent pressure sores on the hips and sacral area.

- Give regular mouth and nose care.

Observing and Reporting
Tube Feedings

Report any of these to the nurse:

- mouth or nose sores

- shortness of breath

- difficulty breathing

- pale or blue-tinged skin

- nausea

- vomiting

- choking

- abdominal cramping

- the resident pulling on the tube

- redness or drainage near the opening

- feeding pump alarm sounds (report to the nurse immediately)

Unit 10. Describe how to assist residents with special needs

Many devices can help people who are recovering from or adapting to a physical condition to feed themselves. These devices are called adaptive equipment or assistive devices. These include special plates, cups, and utensils. In addition to the cues you learned about earlier, residents may use other special dining techniques.

For visually-impaired residents:

- Face the resident when speaking and use a normal tone of voice.

- Read the meal menu to the resident.

- At mealtime, use the face of an imaginary clock to explain the position of what is in front of them.

- If help is needed, let the resident know when to open her mouth and what food she is eating.

For residents who have had a stroke:

- Place food in the resident's field of vision (Fig. 7-20). A resident may have "blind spots." The nurse will determine a resident's field of vision.

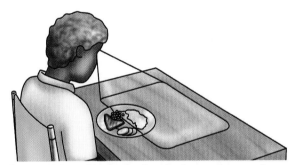

Fig. 7-20. A resident who has had a stroke may have a limited field of vision. Make sure the resident can see what you place in front of him.

- Use assistive devices such as utensils with built-up handle grips, plate guards, and drinking cups. These are ordered for specific residents. They should already be on the tray.

- Watch for signs of choking.

- Serve soft foods if swallowing is difficult.

- Always place food in the unaffected, or non-paralyzed, side of the mouth.

- Make sure the resident swallows the food before offering more bites.

Another resident who may have special needs is a resident with Parkinson's disease. Parkinson's disease is a progressive disease. It causes the brain to degenerate. Progressive and degenerative mean the disease gets worse. It causes greater and greater loss of health and abilities. Parkinson's affects the muscles, causing them to become stiff. It causes stooped posture and a shuffling gait, or walk. Tremors or shaking make it very difficult for a person to eat. For residents who have Parkinson's disease:

- Help them as needed if tremors make it hard for them to eat.

- Place food and drinks close so that the resident can easily reach them.

- Use assistive devices. These promote independence.

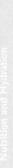

eight
Common, Chronic, and Acute Conditions

Residents in long-term care may have many different diseases and conditions. Diseases and conditions are either acute or chronic. **Acute** means an illness has severe symptoms. An acute illness is short-term. **Chronic** means the disease or condition is long-term or long-lasting. Symptoms are managed. Chronic conditions may have short periods of severity. The person may be hospitalized to stabilize the disease. This book describes diseases or conditions according to the body system in which they are located.

The following is a partial list of the body systems you learned in chapter 4:

- Musculoskeletal
- Nervous
- Circulatory or cardiovascular
- Respiratory
- Urinary
- Gastrointestinal or digestive
- Endocrine
- Reproductive
- Immune and Lymphatic

If you think of the body system under which a disease is classified, the signs and symptoms will be easier to remember. In this chapter, we list only the most common diseases and conditions in long-term care. Pressure sores, a common disorder of the integumentary system, are in chapter 5.

Unit 1. Describe common diseases and disorders of the musculoskeletal system

Arthritis
Arthritis is a general term. It refers to **inflammation**, or swelling, of the joints. It causes stiffness, pain, and decreased mobility. Arthritis may be the result of aging, injury, or an **autoimmune illness**. With an autoimmune illness, the body's immune system attacks normal tissue in the body. There are several types of arthritis.

Osteoarthritis is a common type of arthritis that affects the elderly. It may occur with aging or as the result of joint injury. Hips and knees, which are weight-bearing joints, are usually affected. Joints of the fingers, thumbs, and spine can also be affected. Pain and stiffness seem to increase in cold or damp weather.

Rheumatoid arthritis can affect people of all ages. Joints become inflamed, red, swollen, and very painful. Movement is restricted. Fever, fatigue, and weight loss are also symptoms (Fig. 8-1).

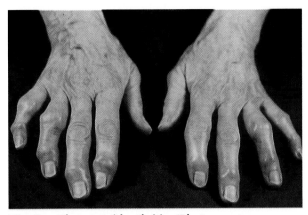

Fig. 8-1. Rheumatoid arthritis. (Photo courtesy Frederick Miller, MD.)

Treatment for arthritis includes:

- anti-inflammatory medications such as aspirin or ibuprofen
- local applications of heat to reduce swelling and pain
- range of motion exercises (chapter 9)
- regular exercise and/or activity routines
- diet to reduce weight or maintain strength

Guidelines
Caring for Residents with Arthritis

- Watch for stomach irritation or heartburn caused by aspirin or ibuprofen. Some residents cannot take these medications. Report signs of stomach irritation or heartburn immediately.

- Encourage activity. Gentle activity can help reduce the effects of arthritis. Follow care plan instructions carefully. Use canes or other aids as needed.

- Adapt activities of daily living (ADLs) to allow independence. Many devices are available to help residents to bathe, dress, and feed themselves even when they have arthritis (chapter 9).

- Choose clothing that is easy to put on and fasten. Encourage use of hand rails and safety bars in the bathroom.

- Treat each resident as an individual. Arthritis is very common among elderly residents. Do not assume that each resident has the same symptoms and needs the same care.

- Help resident's self-esteem. Encourage self-care. Have a positive attitude. Listen to the resident's feelings. You can help him be independent as long as possible.

Osteoporosis

Osteoporosis causes bones to become brittle. Brittle bones can break easily. Weakness in the bones may be due to age, lack of hormones, not enough calcium in bones, alcohol, or lack of exercise. Move residents with osteoporosis very carefully.

Osteoporosis is more common in women after menopause. **Menopause** is the stopping of menstrual periods. Extra calcium and regular exercise can help prevent osteoporosis. Medication, calcium, and fluoride supplements are used to treat osteoporosis. Signs and symptoms of osteoporosis are:

- low back pain
- loss of height
- stooped posture (Fig. 8-2)

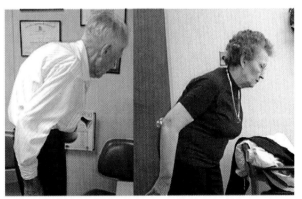

Fig. 8-2. Stooped posture, or "dowager's hump," is a common sign of osteoporosis. (Photos courtesy of Jeffrey T. Behr, MD.)

Fractures and Hip/Knee Replacement

Fractures are broken bones. They are caused by accidents or by osteoporosis.

Preventing falls, which can lead to fractures, is very important. Fractures of arms, elbows, legs, and hips are the most common. Signs and symptoms of a fracture are pain, swelling, bruising, changes in skin color at the site, and limited movement.

Weakened bones make hip fractures more common. A sudden fall can result in a fractured hip. Hip fractures can also occur when weakened bones fracture and cause a fall. A hip fracture is a serious condition. It can take months to heal. Most fractured hips need surgery. Total hip replacement is surgery that replaces the head of the long bone of the leg (femur) where it joins the hip. This is done for these reasons:

- Fractured hip due to an injury or fall which does not heal properly

- Weakened hip due to aging

- Hip is painful and stiff because the joint is weak. The bones are no longer strong enough to bear the person's weight.

The surgery is done through a cut at the hip. An artificial ball-and-socket joint replaces the hip. After the surgery, the resident cannot stand on that leg while the hip heals. A physical therapist will assist after surgery. The goals of care include slowly strengthening the hip muscles and getting the resident walking on that leg.

Be familiar with the resident's care plan. It will state when the resident may begin putting weight on the hip. It will also tell how much the resident is able to do. It is important to help with personal care and using assistive devices, such as walkers or canes.

Guidelines
Hip Replacement

- Keep often-used items, such as medications, telephone, tissues, call light, and water within easy reach. Avoid placing items in high places.

- Dress the affected side first.

- Never rush the resident. Use praise and encouragement. Do this even for small tasks.

- Ask the nurse to give pain medication prior to moving if needed.

- Have the resident sit to do tasks if allowed. This saves energy.

- Follow the care plan exactly, even if the resident wants to do more. Follow orders for weight bearing. An order may be written as partial weight bearing (PWB) or non-weight bearing (NWB). **Partial weight bearing** means the resident is able to support some weight on one or both legs. **Non-weight bearing** means the resident is unable to support any weight on one or both legs. Assist resident as needed with cane, walker, or crutches (chapter 9).

- Never perform ROM exercises on a leg on the side of a hip replacement unless directed by the nurse.

- Caution the resident not to cross legs or turn toes inward. The hip cannot be bent more than 90 degrees. The hip cannot be turned inward (Fig. 8-3).

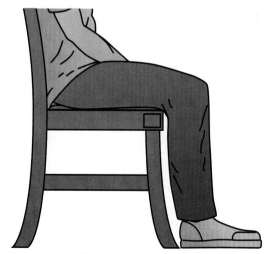

Fig. 8-3. **The hip must maintain a 90-degree angle in the sitting position.**

Observing and Reporting
Hip Replacement

Report any of these to the nurse:

- if the incision is red, draining, bleeding, or warm to the touch

- an increase in pain

- numbness or tingling

- abnormal vital signs, especially change in temperature

- if resident cannot use equipment properly and safely

- if the resident is not following doctor's orders for activity and exercise

- any problems with appetite

Knee replacement is the surgical insertion of a prosthetic knee. This is performed to relieve pain. It also restores motion to a knee damaged by injury or arthritis. It can help stabilize a knee that buckles or gives out repeatedly. Care is similar to that for the hip replacement. However, the recovery time is much shorter. These residents have more ability to care for themselves.

Guidelines
Knee Replacement

- To prevent blood clots, apply special stockings as ordered. One type is a compression stocking. It is a plastic, air-filled, sleeve-like device that is applied to the legs and hooked to a machine. This machine inflates and deflates on its own. It acts in the same way that the muscles usually do under normal activity circumstances. The sleeves are normally applied after surgery while the resident is in bed. Anti-embolic stockings are another type of special stocking. They aid circulation. See later in the chapter for more information on this type of stocking.

- Perform ankle pumps as ordered. These are simple exercises that promote circulation to the legs. Ankle pumps are done by raising the toes and feet toward the ceiling and lowering them again.

- Encourage fluids, especially cranberry and orange juice, which contain Vitamin C, to prevent urinary tract infections (UTIs).

- Assist with deep breathing exercises as ordered.

- Ask the nurse to give pain medication prior to moving and positioning if needed.

Report to the nurse if you notice redness, swelling, heat, or deep tenderness in one or both calves.

Unit 2. Describe common diseases and disorders of the nervous system

Confusion

Confusion is the inability to think clearly. A confused person has trouble focusing his attention and may feel disoriented. Confusion interferes with the ability to make decisions. Personality may change. The person may not know his name, the date, other people, or where he is. Confusion may come on suddenly or gradually. It can be temporary or permanent. A confused person may be angry, depressed, or irritable. Report these symptoms to the nurse. Stay calm. Provide a quiet environment. Speak in a lower tone of voice. Speak clearly and slowly. Introduce yourself each time you see the resident. Remind the resident of his or her location, name, and the date. A calendar can help. Explain what you are going to do. Use simple instructions. Do not rush the resident. Talk to confused residents about plans for the day. Encourage the use of glasses and hearing aids. Make sure they are clean and are not damaged. Keep a routine. Promote self-care and independence. Follow the care plan.

8

Common, Chronic, and Acute Conditions

Dementia

As we age, we may lose some of our ability to think logically and quickly. This ability is called **cognition**. Loss of some of this ability is called cognitive impairment. Cognitive impairment affects concentration and memory. Elderly residents may lose their memories of recent events. This can be frustrating for them. You can help. Encourage them to make lists of things to remember. Write down names and phone numbers. Other normal changes of aging in the brain are slower reaction time, trouble finding or using words, and sleeping less.

Dementia is a more serious loss of mental abilities. It affects thinking, remembering, reasoning, and communicating. As dementia advances, these losses make it hard to perform ADLs such as eating, bathing, dressing, and toileting. **Dementia is not a normal part of aging**.

Causes of dementia include:

- Alzheimer's disease
- Multi-infarct or vascular dementia (a series of strokes that damage the brain)
- Lewy body disease (also called Lewy body dementia)
- Parkinson's disease
- Huntington's disease

Alzheimer's Disease (AD)

Alzheimer's disease (AD) is the most common cause of dementia in the elderly. The National Center for Health Statistics estimates that over half of the people in nursing homes have AD or a related disorder. Alzheimer's disease causes tangled nerve fibers and protein deposits to form in the brain. They eventually cause dementia. The disease gets worse, causing greater and greater loss of health and abilities. The disease cannot be cured. Residents with AD will never recover. They will need more care as the disease progresses.

Symptoms of AD appear gradually. It begins with memory loss. As AD progresses, the symptoms get worse. People with AD may get disoriented. They may be confused about time and place. They can have communication problems. They may lose their ability to read, write, speak, or understand. Mood and behavior changes. Aggressiveness, wandering, and withdrawal are all part of AD. AD progresses to complete loss of all ability to care for oneself.

Each person with AD will show different symptoms at different times. For example, one resident with Alzheimer's may be able to read, but not use the phone or recall her address. Another may have lost the ability to read, but is still able to do simple math. Skills a person has used over a lifetime are usually kept longer (Fig. 8-4).

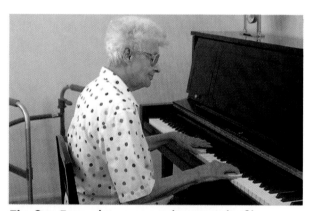

Fig. 8-4. Even when a person loses much of her memory, she may still keep skills she has used her whole life.

Encourage residents with AD to do ADLs. Help them keep their minds and bodies as active as possible. Working, socializing, reading, problem solving, and exercising should all be encouraged (Fig. 8-5). Having them do as much as possible for themselves may even help slow the disease. Look for tasks that are challenging but not frustrating. Help residents succeed in doing them.

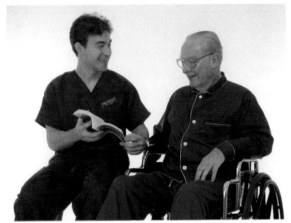

Fig. 8-5. Encourage reading and thinking activities for residents with AD.

Guidelines
Working with Residents with AD

- Do not take their behavior personally.
- Treat residents with AD with dignity and respect, as you would want to be treated.
- Work with the symptoms and behaviors you see.
- Work as a team.
- Encourage communication.
- Take care of yourself.
- Work with family members.
- Follow the goals of the resident care plan.

Guidelines
Communicating with Residents who have AD

- Always approach from the front. Do not startle the resident.
- Determine how close the resident wants you to be.
- Speak in a low, calm voice. Find a room that has very little background noise and distraction.
- Always identify yourself. Use the resident's name. Continue to use the resident's name during the conversation.

- Speak slowly. Use a lower voice than normal. This is calming and easier to understand.
- Repeat yourself, using the same words and phrases, as often as needed.
- Use signs, pictures, gestures, or written words to help communicate.
- Break complex tasks into smaller, simpler ones. Give simple step-by-step instructions as necessary.

Use the same procedures for personal care and ADLs for residents with Alzheimer's disease as with other residents. There are some guidelines to keep in mind when helping residents with AD. Three general principles will help you give the best care:

1. Develop a routine. Stick to it. Being consistent is very important for residents who are confused and easily upset.

2. Promote self-care. Help your residents to care for themselves as much as possible. This will help them cope with this difficult disease.

3. Take good care of yourself, both mentally and physically. This will help you give the best care.

Guidelines
Caring for Residents with AD

- Ensure safety by using non-slip mats, tub seats, and hand-holds.
- Schedule bathing when the resident is least upset. Be organized so the bath can be quick.
- Always use the same steps, explaining them in the same way every time.
- Assist with grooming. Help the people in your care feel attractive and dignified.
- Set up a regular schedule for toileting and follow it.

8

Common, Chronic, and Acute Conditions

180

Unit 2. Describe common diseases and disorders of the nervous system

- Mark the restroom with a sign or a picture as a reminder to use it and where it is.
- Maintain a daily exercise routine.
- Maintain the best nutrition.
- Maintain self-esteem by encouraging independence in ADLs.
- Share in enjoyable activities, looking at pictures, and talking.
- Reward positive and independent behavior with smiles, hugs, and warm touches. Say, "Thank you" often (Fig. 8-6).

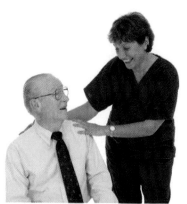

Fig. 8-6. Reward positive behavior with warm touches and smiles.

- Try to identify the causes or "triggers" of agitated behavior. Remove them.

Below are some common difficult behaviors that you may face with Alzheimer's residents. Each resident is different. Work with each person as an individual.

- **Agitation**. Triggers may be a change of routine or caregiver, new or frustrating experiences, or even television. Try to remove triggers. Keep routine constant. Avoid frustration. Focus on a soothing, familiar activity. Try sorting things or looking at pictures. Stay calm. Use a low, soothing voice to speak to and reassure the resident. An arm around the shoulder, patting, or stroking may soothe some residents.

- **Pacing and Wandering**. A resident who walks back and forth in the same area is

pacing. A resident who walks aimlessly around the facility is **wandering**. Restlessness, hunger, disorientation, need for toileting, constipation, pain, forgetting how or where to sit down, need for exercise, or too much daytime napping may cause pacing and wandering (Fig. 8-7). Remove causes when you can. Give nutritious snacks. Encourage an exercise routine. Maintain a toileting schedule. Let residents pace or wander in a safe and secure (locked) area. Keep an eye on them. Suggest another activity, such as going for a walk together.

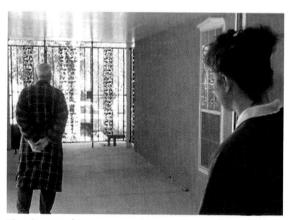

Fig. 8-7. Make sure a resident is in a safe area if he paces or wanders.

- **Hallucinations or Delusions**. A resident who sees things that are not there is having **hallucinations**. A resident who believes things that are not true is having **delusions**. Ignore harmless hallucinations and delusions. Reassure a resident who seems upset or worried. Do not argue with a resident who is imagining things. Do not tease or make fun of the resident. Do not tell the resident that you can see or hear his hallucinations. Redirect resident to other activities or thoughts. Be calm. Reassure resident that you are there to help.

- **Sundowning**. When a person gets restless and agitated in the late afternoon, evening, or night, it is called sundowning. Sundowning may be caused by hunger or fatigue, a change in routine or caregiver, or any new or frustrating situation. Remove triggers. Give snacks or encourage rest. Avoid stressful situations during this time. Limit activities, appointments, trips, and visits. Play soft music. Set a bedtime routine and keep it. Recognize when sundowning occurs. Plan a calming activity just before. Remove caffeine from the diet. Give a soothing back massage. Distract the resident with a simple, calm activity like looking at a magazine. Keep a daily exercise routine.

- **Catastrophic Reactions.** When a person with AD overreacts to something in an unreasonable way, it is called a **catastrophic reaction**. It may be triggered by fatigue, a change of routine or caregiver, or overstimulation (too much noise or activity). It may also be caused by difficult choices or tasks, pain, hunger, or the need for toileting. Respond to catastrophic reactions as you would to agitation or sundowning. For example, remove triggers. Help the resident focus on a soothing activity.

- **Depression.** When residents become withdrawn, lack energy, or do not eat or do things they used to enjoy, they may be depressed. The last unit in this chapter has more information on depression.

Depression may be caused by a loss of independence, the inability to cope, feelings of failure and fear, facing a progressive, incurable illness, or a chemical imbalance.

Report signs of depression to the nurse immediately. It can be treated with medication. Encourage independence, self-care, and activity. Talk about feelings if the resident wishes. Be a good listener. Encourage social interaction.

- **Perseveration or Repetitive Phrasing.** A resident who repeats a word, phrase, question, or activity over and over is **perseverating**. Repeating a word or phrase is also called "repetitive phrasing." This may be caused by disorientation or confusion. Respond to this with patience. Do not try to silence or stop the resident. Answer questions each time they are asked. Use the same words each time.

- **Violent Behavior.** A resident who attacks, hits, or threatens someone is violent. Frustration or overstimulation may trigger violence. It can also be triggered by a change in routine, environment, or caregiver. Look for ways to avoid these triggers. Report any extreme or unusual behavior to the nurse.

If a resident becomes violent, block blows but never hit back (Fig. 8-8). Step out of reach. Call for help if needed. Try to remove triggers. If you are the trigger, step outside to seek help. A resident may respond better to another staff member. Calm resident as you would for agitation or sundowning.

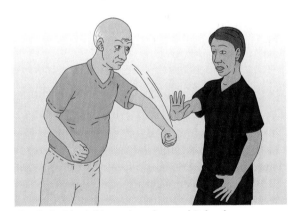

Fig. 8-8. Block blows but do not hit back.

- **Disruptiveness.** Disruptive behavior is anything that disturbs others, such as yelling, banging on furniture, slamming doors, etc. Often this behavior is triggered by a wish for attention, by pain or constipation, or by frustration. Gain the resident's attention. Be calm and friendly. Gently direct the resident to a more private area, if possible. Find out why the behavior is occurring. Ask the resident about it, if possible. There may be a physical reason, such as pain or discomfort.

Notice and praise improvements in behavior. Be tactful and sensitive when you do this. Avoid treating the resident like a child. Tell the resident any changes in schedules, routines, or the environment in advance. Involve the resident in developing routine activities and schedules, if possible. Encourage the resident to join in independent activities that are safe (for example, folding towels). This helps the resident feel in charge. It can prevent feelings of powerlessness. Independence is power. Help the resident find ways to cope. Focus on positive activities he or she may still be able to do, such as knitting, crocheting, crafts, etc. This can provide a diversion.

- **Inappropriate Social Behavior.**
Inappropriate social behavior may be cursing, name calling, or other behavior. As with violent or disruptive behavior, there may be many reasons why a resident is behaving this way. Try not to take it personally. Stay calm. Be reassuring. Try to find out what caused the behavior (for example, too much noise, too many people, too much stress, pain, or discomfort). If possible, gently direct the resident to a private area if he or she is disturbing others. Respond positively to any appropriate behavior. Report any physical abuse or serious verbal abuse to the nurse.

- **Inappropriate Sexual Behavior.**
Inappropriate sexual behavior, such as removing clothes or touching one's own genitals, can embarrass those who see it. Be matter-of-fact when dealing with such behavior. Do not overreact. This may reinforce the behavior. Be sensitive to the nature of the problem. Is the behavior actually intentional? Is it excessive or consistent? Try to distract the resident. If this does not work, gently direct him or her to

a private area. Tell the nurse. A resident may be reacting to a need for physical stimulation or affection. Consider other ways to provide physical stimulation. Try backrubs, a soft doll or stuffed animal to cuddle, comforting blankets, pieces of cloth, or physical touch that is appropriate.

- **Pillaging and Hoarding. Pillaging** is taking things that belong to someone else. A person with dementia may honestly think something belongs to him, even when it clearly does not. **Hoarding** is collecting and putting things away in a guarded way. Pillaging and hoarding should not be considered stealing. A person with Alzheimer's disease cannot and does not steal. Stealing is planned. It requires a conscious effort. In most cases, the person with AD is only collecting something that catches his or her attention. It is common for those with AD to wander in and out of rooms collecting things. They may carry these objects around for a while, and then leave them in other places. This is not intentional. People with AD will often take their own things and leave them in another room, not knowing what they are doing.

You can help lessen problems. Label all personal belongings with the resident's name and room number. This way there is no confusion about what belongs to whom. Place a label, symbol, or object on the resident's door. This helps the resident find his or her own room. Do not tell family that their loved one is "stealing" from others. Prepare the family so they are not upset when they find items that do not belong to their family member. Ask the family to tell staff if they notice strange items in the room. Provide a rummage drawer. This is a drawer with items that are okay and safe for the resident to take with him or her.

Although Alzheimer's disease cannot be cured, there are many ways to improve life for residents with AD.

Reality Orientation is using calendars, clocks, signs, and lists to help residents remember who and where they are. It is useful in early stages of AD when residents are confused but not totally disoriented. In later stages, reality orientation may frustrate residents.

Validation Therapy is letting residents believe they live in the past or in imaginary circumstances. **Validating** means giving value to or approving. Make no attempt to reorient the resident to actual circumstances. Explore the resident's beliefs. Do not argue with or correct them. Validating can give comfort and reduce agitation. It is useful in cases of moderate to severe disorientation.

Reminiscence Therapy is encouraging residents to remember and talk about the past. Explore memories. Ask about details (Fig. 8-9). Focus on a time of life that was pleasant. Work through feelings about a difficult time in the past. It is useful in many stages of AD, but especially with moderate to severe confusion.

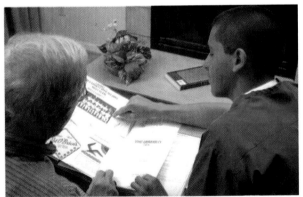

Fig. 8-9. Reminiscence therapy is encouraging a resident to remember and talk about the past.

Activity Therapy uses things residents enjoy to prevent boredom and frustration (Fig. 8-10). These activities also promote self-

esteem. Help the resident take walks, do puzzles, listen to music, or do other things she enjoys. It is useful in most stages of AD.

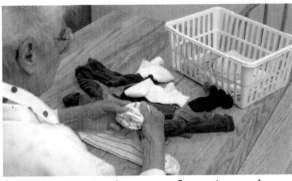

Fig. 8-10. Activities that are not frustrating can be helpful for residents with AD. They promote mental exercise.

Parkinson's Disease

Parkinson's disease is a progressive disease. It causes a section of the brain to degenerate. It affects the muscles, causing them to become stiff. It causes stooped posture and a shuffling **gait**, or walk. It can also cause pill-rolling. This is moving the thumb and first finger together like rolling a pill. Tremors or shaking make it very difficult for a person to do ADLs such as eating and bathing. A person with Parkinson's may have a mask-like facial expression.

Medications may help. Residents are at a high risk for falls. Protect residents from any unsafe areas and conditions. Help with ADLs as needed. Assist with range of motion exercises to prevent contractures and to strengthen muscles. Encourage self-care. Be patient with self-care and communication.

Multiple Sclerosis (MS)

Multiple sclerosis is a progressive disease. It affects the central nervous system. When a person has MS, the protective covering for the nerves, spinal cord, and white matter of the brain breaks down over time. Without this covering, or sheath, nerves cannot send messages to and from the brain in a normal way. Residents with MS have varying abilities. Symptoms include blurred vision, fatigue, tremors, poor balance, and trouble walking. Weakness, numbness, tingling, incontinence, and behavior changes are also symptoms. MS can cause blindness, contractures (chapter 9), and loss of function in the arms and legs.

Be patient with self-care and movement. Help with ADLs. Allow enough time for tasks. Offer rest periods as necessary. Give resident plenty of time to communicate. Do not rush him or her. Prevent falls, which may be due to a lack of coordination, fatigue, and vision problems. Stress can worsen the effects of MS. Be calm. Listen to residents when they want to talk. Encourage proper diet. Offer plenty of fluids. Give excellent skin care to prevent pressure sores. Assist with range of motion exercises to prevent contractures and to strengthen muscles.

CVA or Stroke

The medical term for a stroke is a cerebrovascular accident (CVA). CVA, or stroke, is caused when blood supply to the brain is cut off suddenly by a clot or a ruptured blood vessel (Fig. 8-11). Without blood, part of the brain gets no oxygen. Brain cells die. Brain tissue is further damaged by leaking blood, clots, and swelling. See chapter 2 for more information on the warning signs of a stroke.

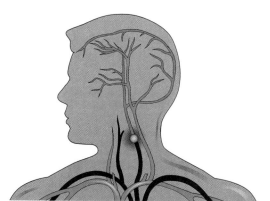

Fig. 8-11. A stroke is caused when the blood supply to the brain is cut off suddenly by a clot or ruptured blood vessel.

The two sides of the brain control different functions. Symptoms depend on which side of the brain the stroke affected. Weaknesses on the right side show that the left side of the brain was affected. Weaknesses on the left side show that the right side of the brain was affected.

Strokes can be mild or severe. Afterward, a resident may experience any of these problems:

- weakness on one side of the body, called **hemiparesis**

- paralysis on one side of the body, called **hemiplegia**

- tendency to ignore a weak or paralyzed side of the body

- inability to speak or speak clearly, called **aphasia**

- inability to express needs to others through speech or writing, called expressive aphasia

- trouble understanding spoken or written words

- loss of sensations, such as temperature or touch

- loss of bowel or bladder control

- confusion

- laughing or crying without any reason, or when it is inappropriate, called **emotional lability**

- poor judgment

- memory loss

- loss of thinking and learning abilities

- trouble swallowing, called dysphagia

If the stroke was mild, the resident may experience few, if any, of these complications. Physical therapy may help regain physical abilities. Speech and occupational therapy can also help a person learn to communicate and perform ADLs again.

Guidelines
Residents Recovering from Stroke

A resident with paralysis, weakness, or loss of movement will usually have physical or occupational therapy. Residents may also perform leg exercises to aid circulation. Safety is very important when residents are exercising.

- Adapt procedures when providing personal care for residents with one-sided paralysis or weakness. Carefully assist with shaving, grooming, and bathing.

- When helping with transfers or walking, stand on the weaker side. Support the weaker side. Lead with the stronger side (Fig. 8-12). Always use a gait belt for safety.

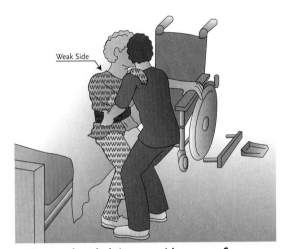

Weak Side

Fig. 8-12. When helping a resident transfer, support the weak side while leading with the stronger side.

- Never refer to the weaker side as the "bad side." Do not talk about the "bad" leg or arm. Use the terms "weaker" or "involved" to refer to the side with paralysis.

- If residents have a loss of touch or sensation, check for potentially harmful situations (for example, heat and sharp objects). If residents are unable to sense or move part of the body, check and change positioning to prevent pressure sores.

- Residents with speech loss or communication problems may receive speech therapy. You may be asked to help. This may in-

clude helping residents recognize written words or spoken words. Speech therapists will also evaluate a resident's swallowing ability. They will decide if swallowing therapy or thickened liquids are needed.

- Confusion and memory loss are upsetting. Residents often cry for no reason after suffering a stroke. Be very patient and understanding. Keep a routine of care. This helps residents feel more secure.

Here are ways to help residents recovering from stroke:

- Encourage independence and self-esteem. Let the resident do things for herself whenever possible even if you could do a better or faster job.

- Make tasks less difficult for residents.

- Notice and praise residents' efforts to do things for themselves even when they are unsuccessful.

- Praise even the smallest successes. This builds confidence.

Guidelines
Dressing a Resident with One-Sided Weakness

- Dress weaker side first. Place the weaker arm or leg into the clothing. This prevents unnecessary bending and stretching of the limb. Undress stronger side first. Lead with the stronger side. Then remove weaker arm or leg from clothing to prevent the limb from being stretched and twisted.

- Provide adaptive equipment to help resident dress himself.

- Encourage self-care.

Guidelines
Communicating with Residents Who Have Had a Stroke

Depending on the severity of the stroke and speech loss or confusion, these tips may help:

8

Common, Chronic, and Acute Conditions

- Keep questions and directions simple.

- Phrase questions so they can be answered with a "yes" or "no."

- Agree on signals, such as shaking or nodding the head, or raising a hand or finger for "yes" or "no."

- Give residents time to respond. Listen attentively.

- Use a pencil and paper if a resident can write. A thick handle or tape around it may help the resident hold it more easily.

- Use pictures, gestures, or pointing. Use communication boards or special cards to aid communication (Fig. 8-13).

A	B	C	D	E	F	G	H	I	J	K	L	M
N	O	P	Q	R	S	T	U	V	W	X	Y	Z

1	2	3	4	5	6
7	8	9	10	11	12
13	14	15	16	17	18
19	20	21	22	23	24
25	26	27	28	29	30

CALL BELL	BED UP	BED DOWN	UP IN CHAIR
DOCTOR	NURSE	HUSBAND/SON	WIFE/DAUGHTER
ICE/WATER	MILK	BATHROOM	BEDPAN
RAZOR/SHAVE	GLASSES	MEDICINE	WATCH/TIME
WHEELCHAIR	BACK TO BED	TOO HOT	TOO COLD
CLERGY	HUNGRY	DRINK	TEA/COFFEE
URINAL	BRUSH TEETH	TISSUES	COMB/BRUSH
PEN/PAPER	TELEPHONE	RADIO/TV	MAGAZINE/NEWSPAPER

Fig. 8-13. **A sample communication board.**

- Keep the call signal within reach of residents. They can let you know when you are needed.

Guidelines for assisting a person recovering from stroke with eating are in chapter 7.

Never talk about residents as if they were not there. Just because they cannot speak does not mean they cannot hear. Treat all residents with respect.

Head and Spinal Cord Injuries

Diving, sports injuries, falls, car and motorcycle accidents, industrial accidents, war, and criminal violence are some causes of these injuries. Head injuries can cause permanent brain damage. Spinal cord injuries depend on the force of impact and where the spine is injured. The higher the injury, the greater the loss of function. People with head and spinal cord injuries may have **paraplegia**. This is a loss of function of lower body and legs. These injuries may also cause **quadriplegia**. The person is then unable to use his legs, trunk, and arms (Fig. 8-14).

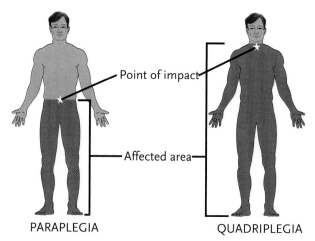

PARAPLEGIA   QUADRIPLEGIA

Fig. 8-14.

Guidelines
Head or Spinal Cord Injury

- Give emotional support, as well as physical help.

- Be patient with all care.

- Safety is very important. Be very careful that residents do not fall or burn themselves. Because these residents have no sensation, they cannot feel a burn.

- Give good skin care to prevent pressure sores.

- Assist residents to change positions at least every two hours to prevent pressure sores. Be gentle when repositioning.

- Perform passive range of motion exercises as ordered to prevent contractures and to strengthen muscles.

- Allow as much independence as possible with ADLs.

- Immobility leads to constipation. Encourage fluids and proper diet (high in fiber), if ordered.

- Loss of ability to empty the bladder may lead to the need for a catheter. Urinary tract infections are common. Encourage a high intake of fluids and give extra catheter care as needed.

- Lack of activity leads to poor circulation and fatigue. You may be directed to use special stockings to increase circulation.

- Offer rest periods as necessary.

- Difficulty coughing and shallow breathing can lead to pneumonia. Encourage deep breathing exercises as ordered.

- Male residents may have involuntary erections. These are not deliberate. Provide for privacy and be sensitive to this.

- Assist with bowel and bladder training if needed.

Unit 3. Describe common diseases and disorders of the circulatory system

High Blood Pressure (Hypertension)
When blood pressure is consistently 140/90 or higher, a person is diagnosed as having hypertension, or high blood pressure. If blood pressure is between 120/80 and 139/89 mmHg, it is called prehypertension. The person does not have high blood pressure now but is likely to develop it in the future.

A hardening and narrowing of the blood vessels causes high blood pressure (Fig. 8-15). It can also result from kidney disease, tumors of the adrenal gland, and pregnancy. High blood pressure can develop in persons of any age.

Signs and symptoms of high blood pressure are not always obvious. This is especially true in the early stages. Often it is only discovered when blood pressure is taken. Persons may complain of headache, blurred vision, and dizziness.

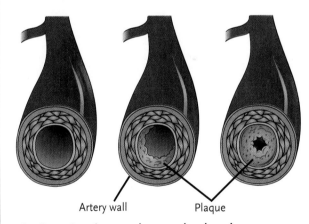

Artery wall   Plaque

Fig. 8-15. **Arteries may become hardened, or narrower, because of a buildup of plaque. Hardened arteries cause high blood pressure.**

Guidelines
High Blood Pressure

- High blood pressure can lead to serious problems such as CVA, heart attack, kidney disease, or blindness. Treatment to control it is vital. Residents may take diuretics or medication that lowers cholesterol. **Diuretics** are drugs that reduce fluid in the body.

8

Common, Chronic, and Acute Conditions

- Residents may also have a prescribed exercise program or be on a special low-fat, low-sodium diet. Encourage residents to follow their diet and exercise programs.

Heart Attack or Myocardial Infarction

When blood flow to the heart muscle is completely blocked, oxygen and nutrients fail to reach the cells in that region (Fig. 8-16). Waste products are not removed. The muscle cell dies. This is called a heart attack or myocardial infarction (MI). See chapter 2 for warning signs of a heart attack.

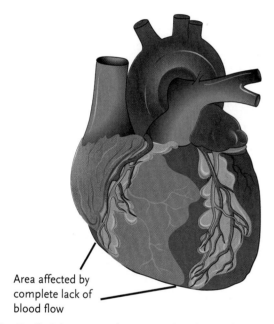

Area affected by complete lack of blood flow

Fig. 8-16. A heart attack occurs when blood flow to the heart or a portion of the heart is cut off completely.

Guidelines
Heart Attack

- Most residents will be placed on a regular exercise program.

- Residents may be on a diet that is low in fat and cholesterol and/or a low-sodium diet.

- Medications may be used to regulate heart rate and blood pressure.

- Quitting smoking will be encouraged.

- A stress management program may be started to help reduce stress levels.

- Residents recovering from a heart attack may need to avoid cold temperatures.

Coronary Artery Disease (CAD)

Coronary artery disease occurs when the blood vessels in the coronary arteries narrow. This reduces the supply of blood to the heart muscle and deprives it of oxygen and nutrients. Over time, as fatty deposits block the artery, the muscle that was supplied by the blood vessel dies. CAD can lead to heart attack or stroke.

The heart muscle that is not getting enough oxygen causes chest pain, or **angina pectoris**. The heart needs more oxygen during exercise, stress, excitement, or a heavy meal. In CAD, narrow blood vessels keep the extra blood with oxygen from getting to the heart (Fig. 8-17).

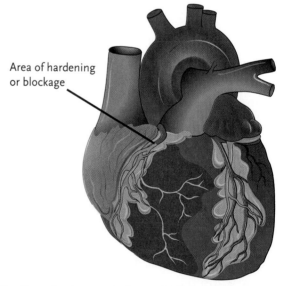

Area of hardening or blockage

Fig. 8-17. Angina pectoris results from the heart not getting enough oxygen.

The pain of angina pectoris is usually described as pressure or tightness. It occurs in the left side or the center of the chest behind the sternum or breastbone. Some people have pain moving down the inside of the left arm or to the neck and left side of the jaw. A person suffering from angina pectoris may sweat or look pale. The person may feel dizzy and have trouble breathing.

Guidelines
Angina Pectoris

- Rest is extremely important. Rest reduces the heart's need for extra oxygen. It helps the blood flow return to normal, often within three to fifteen minutes.

- Medication is also needed to relax the walls of the coronary arteries. This allows them to open and get more blood to the heart. This medication, nitroglycerin, is a small tablet that the resident places under the tongue. There it dissolves and is rapidly absorbed. Residents who have angina pectoris may keep nitroglycerin on hand to use as symptoms arise. Nursing assistants are not allowed to give any medication unless they have had special training. Tell the nurse if a resident needs help taking the medication. Nitroglycerin also is available as a patch. Do not remove the patch. Tell the nurse immediately if the patch comes off.

- Residents may also need to avoid heavy meals, overeating, intense exercise, and cold or hot and humid weather.

Congestive Heart Failure (CHF)

Coronary artery disease, heart attack, high blood pressure, or other disorders may damage the heart. When the heart muscle has been severely damaged, it fails to pump effectively. Blood backs up into the heart instead of circulating. This is called congestive heart failure, or CHF. It can occur on one or both sides of the heart.

Observing and Reporting
CHF

- trouble breathing; coughing or gurgling with breathing

- dizziness, confusion, and fainting

- pale or blue skin

- low blood pressure

- swelling of the feet and ankles (edema)

- bulging veins in the neck

- weight gain

Guidelines
CHF

- Medications can strengthen the heart muscle and improve its pumping.

- Medications help remove excess fluids. This means more trips to the bathroom. Answer call lights promptly.

- A low-sodium diet or a fluid restriction may be prescribed.

- A weakened heart pump may make it hard for residents to walk, carry items, or climb stairs. Limited activity or bed rest may be prescribed.

- Intake and output of fluids may need to be measured.

- Resident may be weighed daily at the same time to note weight gain from fluid retention.

- Elastic leg stockings may be applied to reduce swelling in feet and ankles (see procedure on next page).

- Range of motion exercises improve muscle tone when activity and exercise are limited (Fig. 8-18). See chapter 9 for range of motion information.

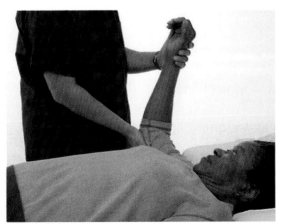

Fig. 8-18. Range of motion exercises improve muscle tone.

- Extra pillows may help residents who have trouble breathing. Keeping the head of the bed elevated may also help with breathing.

- Help with personal care and ADLs as needed.

Peripheral Vascular Disease (PVD)

Peripheral vascular disease is a condition in which the legs, feet, arms or hands do not have enough blood circulation. This is due to fatty deposits in the blood vessels that harden over time. Signs and symptoms include:

- cool or cold arms and legs

- swelling in hands or feet

- pale or bluish hands or feet (cyanosis)

- bluish nail beds

- ulcers of legs or feet

Some changes in health may lead to inactivity. A lack of mobility may contribute to PVD. For some cases of poor circulation to legs and feet, elastic stockings are ordered. These special stockings help prevent swelling and blood clots. They aid circulation. These stockings are called anti-embolic hose. They need to be put on before the resident gets out of bed. Follow manufacturer's instructions and illustrations on how to put them on.

Putting a knee-high elastic stocking on a resident

Equipment: elastic stockings

1. **Wash hands.**

   Provides for infection control.

2. **Identify yourself by name. Identify resident by name.**

   Resident has right to know identity of his or her caregiver. Addressing resident by name shows respect and establishes correct identification.

3. **Explain procedure to resident. Speak clearly, slowly, and directly. Maintain face-to-face contact whenever possible.**

   Promotes understanding and independence.

4. **Provide for resident's privacy with curtain, screen, or door.**

   Maintains resident's right to privacy and dignity.

5. **Turn stocking inside-out at least to heel area (Fig. 8-19).**

   Allows stocking to roll on gently.

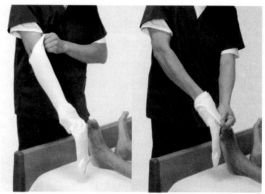

Fig. 8-19.

6. **Gently place foot of stocking over toes, foot, and heel (Fig. 8-20).**

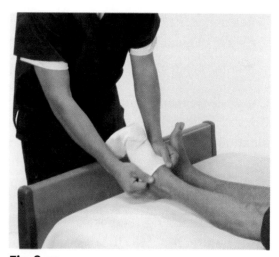

Fig. 8-20.

7. **Gently pull top of stocking over foot, heel, and leg.**

   Being gentle promotes resident's comfort and safety. Avoid force and over-extending joints.

8. **Make sure there are no twists or wrinkles in stocking after it is on (Fig 8-21). It must fit smoothly.**

   Twists or wrinkles cause the stocking to be too tight, reducing circulation.

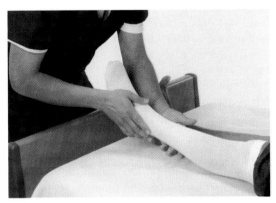

Fig. 8-21.

9. **Remove privacy measures.**

10. **Before leaving, place call light within resident's reach.**

    Allows resident to communicate with staff as necessary.

11. **Wash hands.**

    Provides for infection control.

12. **Report any changes in resident to nurse.**

    Provides nurse with information to assess resident.

13. **Document procedure using facility guidelines.**

    What you write is a legal record of what you did. If you don't document it, legally it didn't happen.

✎ *You must place the stocking over toes and heel correctly. This makes it easier to bring it up the leg smoothly. Do not force the stocking over the foot.*

Unit 4. **Describe common diseases and disorders of the respiratory system**

COPD

Chronic obstructive pulmonary disease (COPD) refers to a number of chronic lung disorders that obstruct the airways. COPD is a chronic disease. The resident may live for years with it but never be cured. Residents with COPD have difficulty breathing, especially in getting air out of the lungs. The most common form of COPD is a combination of chronic bronchitis and emphysema.

Over time, a resident with either of these lung disorders becomes chronically ill and weakened. There is a high risk for acute lung infections, such as pneumonia. Pneumonia can be caused by a bacterial, viral, or fungal infection. Acute inflammation occurs in lung tissue. The affected person develops a high fever, chills, cough, chest pains, and rapid pulse. It is usually treated with antibiotics and other medications to reduce congestion and inflammation. Recovery may take longer for older adults and persons with chronic illnesses.

Sometimes medications for lung conditions are given directly into the lungs by sprays or inhalers (Fig. 8-22).

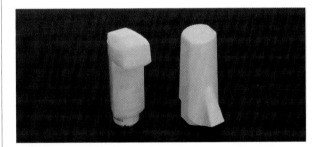

Fig. 8-22. An inhaler.

When the lungs and brain do not get enough oxygen, all body systems are affected. Residents may have a constant fear of not being able to breathe. This can cause them to sit upright to improve their ability to expand the lungs. These residents can have poor appetites. They usually do not get enough sleep. All of this can add to feelings of weakness and poor health. They may feel they have lost control of their bodies, and particularly their breathing. They may fear suffocation.

Residents with COPD may have these symptoms:

- chronic cough or wheeze
- trouble breathing, especially with inhaling and exhaling deeply

- shortness of breath, especially during physical effort
- pale or blue skin (cyanosis) or reddish-purple skin
- confusion
- general state of weakness
- trouble completing meals due to shortness of breath
- fear and anxiety

Guidelines
COPD

- Colds or viruses can make residents very ill quickly. Always observe and report signs of symptoms getting worse.
- Help residents sit upright or lean forward. Offer pillows for support (Fig. 8-23).

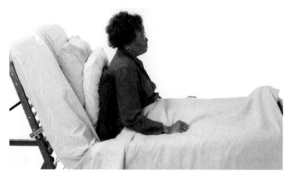

Fig. 8-23. It helps residents with COPD to sit upright and lean forward slightly.

- Offer plenty of fluids and small, frequent meals.
- Encourage a well-balanced diet.
- Keep oxygen supply available as ordered.
- Be calm and supportive. Being unable to breathe or fearing suffocation is very frightening.
- Use good infection control. Encourage handwashing and the disposal of used tissues.
- Encourage as much independence with ADLs as possible.
- Remind residents to avoid exposure to infections, especially colds and the flu.

- Ensure that residents always have help available, especially in case of a breathing crisis.
- Encourage pursed-lip breathing. Pursed-lip breathing is placing the lips as if kissing and taking controlled breaths. A nurse should teach residents how to do this type of breathing.
- Encourage residents to save energy for important tasks. Encourage residents to rest.

Observing and Reporting
COPD

Report any of these to the nurse:

- temperature over 101°F
- changes in breathing patterns, including shortness of breath
- changes in color or consistency of lung secretions
- changes in mental state or personality
- refusal to take medications
- excessive weight loss
- increasing dependence upon caregivers and family

Unit 5. Describe common diseases and disorders of the urinary system

Urinary Tract Infection (UTI)

UTIs cause inflammation of the bladder and the ureters. This causes burning during urination. It also causes a frequent feeling of needing to urinate. UTIs may be caused by bacterial infection. Being bed-bound can cause urine to stay in the bladder too long. This helps bacteria to grow.

UTIs are more common in women. The urethra is much shorter in women (three to four inches) than in men (seven to eight inches). Bacteria can reach a woman's bladder more easily.

8

Common, Chronic, and Acute Conditions

Guidelines
Preventing UTIs

- Encourage female residents to wipe from front to back after elimination (Fig. 8-24). When you give perineal care, make sure you do this as well.

- Give good perineal care when changing adult briefs.

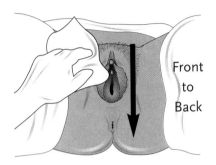

Fig. 8-24. After elimination, women need to wipe from front to back to prevent infection.

- Encourage plenty of fluids. Drinking 2-3 glasses of cranberry or blueberry juice daily acidifies urine. This helps to prevent infection. Vitamin C also has this effect.

- Offer bedpan or a trip to the toilet at least every two hours. Answer call lights promptly.

- Taking showers, rather than baths, helps prevent UTIs.

- Report cloudy, dark, or foul-smelling urine, or if a resident urinates often and in small amounts.

Unit 6. Describe common diseases and disorders of the gastrointestinal system

Constipation, a GI disorder, is discussed in chapter 5. Information on hepatitis is in chapter 2.

Hemorrhoids

Hemorrhoids are enlarged veins in the rectum. They may also be visible outside the anus. Rectal itching, burning, pain, and bleeding are symptoms of hemorrhoids. Treatment may include medications, compresses, and special baths. Surgery may be necessary. When cleaning the anus, take care to avoid causing pain and bleeding from hemorrhoids.

Diarrhea

Diarrhea is frequent elimination of liquid or semi-liquid feces. Abdominal cramps, urgency, nausea, and vomiting can accompany diarrhea, depending on the cause. Infections, microorganisms, irritating foods, and medications can cause diarrhea. Treatment is usually medication and a change of diet. A diet of bananas, rice, apples, and tea/toast (BRAT diet) is often suggested.

Gastroesophageal Reflux Disease (GERD)

Gastroesophageal reflux disease, commonly referred to as GERD, is a chronic condition in which the liquid contents of the stomach back up into the esophagus. The liquid can inflame and damage the lining of the esophagus. It can cause bleeding or ulcers. In addition, scars from tissue damage can narrow the esophagus and make swallowing difficult.

Heartburn is the most common symptom of GERD. Heartburn and GERD must be reported. These conditions are usually treated with medications. Serving the evening meal three to four hours before bedtime may increase comfort. Give the resident an extra pillow so the body is more upright during sleep. Ask the resident not to lay down until at least two hours after eating. Serving the largest meal of the day at lunchtime, serving several small meals throughout the day, and reducing fast foods, fatty foods, and spicy foods may help. Stopping smoking, not drinking alcohol, and wearing loose-fitting clothes may also help.

Ostomy

An **ostomy** is an operation to create an opening from an area inside the body to the outside. The terms "colostomy" and "ileostomy" refer to the surgical removal of a portion of the intestines. It may be necessary due to bowel disease, cancer, or trauma. (More information on cancer is listed later in the chapter.) In a resident with one of these ostomies, the end of the intestine is brought out of the body through an artificial opening in the abdomen. This opening is called a **stoma**. Stool, or feces, are eliminated through the ostomy rather than through the anus.

The terms "colostomy" and "ileostomy" tell what section of the intestine was removed and the type of stool that will be eliminated. In a colostomy, stool will generally be semisolid. With an ileostomy, stool may be liquid. It may be irritating to the skin.

Residents who have had an ostomy wear a disposable bag that fits over the stoma to collect the feces (Fig. 8-25). The bag is attached to the skin by adhesive. A belt may also be used to secure it. Many people manage the ostomy appliance by themselves. If you are providing ostomy care, make certain the resident receives good skin care and hygiene. Empty or replace the ostomy bag whenever a stool is eliminated. Always wear gloves and wash hands carefully. Teach proper handwashing to residents with ostomies.

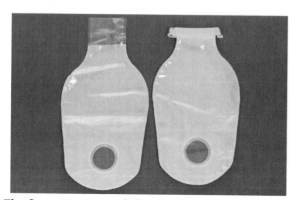

Fig. 8-25. An open and closed ostomy bag.

Residents with ostomies may feel they have lost control of a basic function. They may be embarrassed or angry. Be sensitive. Be supportive. Provide privacy for ostomy care.

Caring for an ostomy

Equipment: disposable bed protector, bath blanket, clean ostomy bag and belt/appliance, toilet paper, basin of warm water, soap or cleanser, washcloth, skin cream as ordered, 2 towels, plastic disposable bag, gloves

1. **Wash hands.**
   Provides for infection control.

2. **Identify yourself to resident by name. Address resident by name.**
   Resident has right to know identity of his or her caregiver. Addressing resident by name shows respect and establishes correct identification.

3. **Explain procedure to resident, speaking clearly, slowly, and directly, maintaining face-to-face contact whenever possible.**
   Promotes understanding and independence.

4. **Provide for resident's privacy during procedure with curtain, screen, or door.**
   Maintains resident's right to privacy and dignity.

5. **Adjust bed to a safe working level.**
   Prevents injury to you and to resident.

6. **Place protective sheet under resident. Cover resident with a bath blanket. Pull down the top sheet and blankets. Only expose ostomy site. Offer resident a towel to keep clothing dry.**
   Maintains resident's right to privacy and dignity.

7. **Put on gloves.**
   Provides for infection control.

8. **Remove ostomy bag carefully. Place it in plastic bag. Note the color, odor, consistency, and amount of stool in the bag.**
   Changes in stool can indicate a problem.

9. **Wipe area around stoma with toilet paper. Discard the paper in plastic bag (Fig. 8-26).**

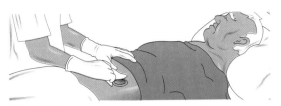

Fig. 8-26.

10. **Using a washcloth and warm soapy water, wash the area in one direction, away from the stoma. Pat dry with another towel. Apply cream as ordered.**
Keeping skin clean and dry prevents skin breakdown.

11. **Place the clean ostomy appliance on resident. Make sure the bottom of the bag is clamped.**

12. **Remove disposable bed protector and discard. Place soiled linens in proper container.**

13. **Remove bag. Discard the bag in the proper container.**

14. **Remove and dispose of gloves properly.**

15. **Return bed to appropriate level. Place call light within resident's reach.**
Lowering the bed provides for safety. Signaling device allows resident to communicate with staff as necessary.

16. **Wash hands.**
Provides for infection control.

17. **Report any changes in resident to the nurse.**
Provides nurse with information to assess resident.

18. **Document procedure according to facility guidelines.**
What you write is a legal record of what you did. If you don't document it, legally it didn't happen.

Unit 7. Describe common diseases and disorders of the endocrine system

Diabetes

Diabetes mellitus is commonly called **diabetes**. Diabetes is a disease in which the body does not produce enough or properly use insulin. **Insulin** is a hormone that converts glucose, or natural sugar, into energy for the body. Without insulin to process glucose, these sugars collect in the blood. This causes circulation problems and can damage vital organs. Diabetes is common in people with a family history of the illness, in the elderly, and people who are obese. Two major types of diabetes are:

1. **Type 1 diabetes** is usually diagnosed in children and young adults. It was formerly known as juvenile diabetes. It most often appears before age 20. In Type 1 diabetes, the body does not produce enough insulin. The condition will continue throughout a person's life. A person can develop Type 1 diabetes up to age 40. Type 1 diabetes is treated with insulin and diet.

2. **Type 2 diabetes** is the most common form of diabetes. In Type 2 diabetes, either the body does not produce enough insulin or the body fails to properly use insulin. This is known as "insulin resistance." It can usually be controlled with diet and/or oral medications. It is also called adult-onset diabetes. Type 2 diabetes usually develops slowly. It is the milder form of diabetes. It typically develops after age 35. The risk of getting it increases with age. However, the number of children with Type 2 diabetes is growing rapidly. Type 2 diabetes often occurs in obese people or those with a family history of the disease.

Other types of diabetes are:

Pre-diabetes occurs when a person's blood glucose levels are above normal but not high enough for a diagnosis of Type 2 diabetes. Research indicates that some damage to the body, especially the heart and circulatory system, may already be occurring during pre-diabetes.

Pregnant women who have never had diabetes before but who have high blood sugar (glucose) levels during pregnancy are said to have **gestational diabetes**.

People with diabetes may have these signs and symptoms (Fig. 8-27):

- excessive thirst
- extreme hunger
- weight loss
- high levels of blood sugar
- sugar in the urine
- frequent urination
- sudden vision changes
- tingling or numbness in hands or feet
- feeling very tired much of the time
- very dry skin
- sores that are slow to heal
- more infections than usual

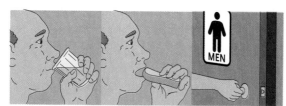

Fig. 8-27. Increased thirst, hunger, and urination are all symptoms of diabetes.

Diabetes can lead to further complications:

- Changes in the circulatory system can cause heart attack and stroke, reduced circulation, poor wound healing, and kidney and nerve damage.
- Damage to the eyes can cause vision loss and blindness.
- Poor circulation and impaired wound healing may cause leg and foot ulcers, infected wounds, and gangrene. Gangrene can lead to amputation.

- Insulin shock and diabetic coma can be life-threatening. See chapter 2 for more information on insulin shock and diabetic coma. Discuss each individual resident's status with the nurse.

Diabetes must be carefully controlled to prevent complications and severe illness. When working with people with diabetes, follow care plan instructions carefully.

Guidelines
Diabetes

- As discussed in chapter 7, a person with diabetes must follow diet instructions exactly. The intake of carbohydrates, including breads, potatoes, grains, pasta, and sugars, must be monitored. Meals must be eaten at the same time each day. The resident must eat all that is served. If a resident will not eat what is served, or if you suspect that he or she is not following the diet, tell the nurse.

- Encourage the right portions of healthy foods. This includes foods that have less salt and fat.

- Encourage the person to exercise. A regular exercise program is important. Exercise affects how quickly bodies use food. Exercise also improves circulation. Exercises may include walking or other active exercise (Fig. 8-28). Help with exercise as necessary. Try to make it fun. A walk can be a chore or it can be the highlight of the day.

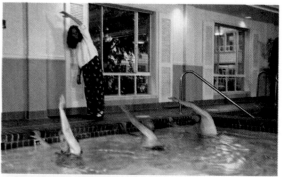

Fig. 8-28. Exercise programs are very important for diabetic residents.

- Observe the resident's management of insulin. Doses are calculated exactly. They are given at the same time each day. Nursing assistants should know when residents take insulin and when their meals should be served. There must be a balance between the insulin level and food intake. Unless you have had special training, you will not inject insulin.

- Perform urine and blood tests only as directed (Fig. 8-29). Sometimes the care plan will specify a daily blood or urine test for sugar or insulin levels. Not all states allow you to do this. Know your state's rules. Perform tests only as directed and allowed.

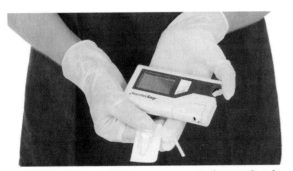

Fig. 8-29. This equipment measures glucose levels in the blood.

- Give foot care as directed. Poor circulation occurs in diabetics. Even a small sore on the leg or foot can grow into a large wound. It can require amputation. Careful foot care, including regular, daily inspection, is vital. The goals of diabetic foot care are to check for irritation or sores, to promote blood circulation, and to prevent infection.

- Encourage diabetics to wear comfortable, well-fitting leather shoes that do not hurt their feet. Leather shoes breathe and help prevent buildup of moisture. To avoid injuries to the feet, diabetics should never go barefoot. White cotton socks are best to absorb sweat. You should never trim or clip any resident's toenails, but especially not a diabetic's toenails. Only a nurse or doctor should do this.

Unit 8. Describe common diseases and disorders of the reproductive system

Vaginitis

Vaginitis is an infection of the vagina. It may be caused by a bacteria, protozoa (one-celled animals), or fungus (yeast). It may also be caused by hormonal changes after menopause. Women who have vaginitis have a white vaginal discharge. This is accompanied by itching and burning. Report these symptoms to the nurse.

Benign Prostatic Hypertrophy (BPH)

Benign prostatic hypertrophy is a disorder that occurs in men as they age. The prostate becomes enlarged. This causes pressure on the urethra. The pressure leads to problems urinating and/or emptying the bladder. Benign prostatic hypertrophy is treated with medications or surgery. A test is available to screen for cancer of the prostate. As men age, they are at increased risk for prostate cancer. Prostate cancer is usually slow-growing. It is responsive to treatment if caught early.

Unit 9. Describe common diseases and disorders of the immune and lymphatic systems

HIV and AIDS

Acquired immunodeficiency syndrome (AIDS) is caused by the human immunodeficiency virus (HIV). HIV attacks the body's immune system and gradually disables it. The HIV-infected person has less resistance to other infections. Death results from these infections. However, medications help people live longer. HIV is a sexually-transmitted disease. It is also spread through the blood, infected needles, or to the fetus from its mother.

In general, HIV affects the body in stages. The first stage shows symptoms like the flu, with fever, muscle aches, cough, and fatigue. These are signs of the immune system fighting the infection. As the infection worsens, the immune system overreacts. It attacks not only the virus, but also normal tissue.

When the virus weakens the immune system in later stages, a group of problems may appear. These include infections, tumors, and central nervous system symptoms. These would not occur if the immune system were healthy. This stage of the disease is known as AIDS.

In the late stages of AIDS, damage to the central nervous system may cause memory loss, poor coordination, paralysis, and confusion. These symptoms together are known as AIDS dementia complex.

These are the signs and symptoms of HIV infection and AIDS:

- appetite loss
- involuntary weight loss of ten pounds or more
- vague, flu-like symptoms, including fever, cough, weakness, and severe or constant fatigue
- night sweats
- swollen lymph nodes in the neck, underarms, or groin
- severe diarrhea
- dry cough
- skin rashes
- painful white spots in the mouth or on the tongue
- cold sores or fever blisters on the lips and flat, white ulcers on a reddened base in the mouth
- cauliflower-like warts on the skin and in the mouth
- inflamed and bleeding gums
- bruising that does not go away
- low resistance to infection, particularly pneumonia, but also tuberculosis, herpes, bacterial infections, and hepatitis
- Kaposi's sarcoma, a form of skin cancer that appears as purple or red skin lesions (Fig. 8-30)

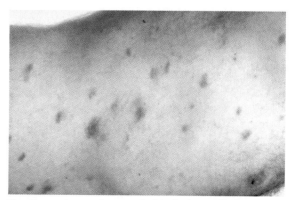

Fig. 8-30. A purple or red skin lesion called Kaposi's sarcoma can be a sign of AIDS.

- AIDS dementia complex

Infections, such as pneumonia, tuberculosis, or hepatitis, invade the body when the immune system is weak and cannot defend itself. These illnesses worsen AIDS. They further weaken the immune system. It is hard to treat these infections. Generally, over time, a person develops a resistance to some antibiotics. These infections often cause death in people with AIDS.

Persons with HIV are treated with drugs that slow the progress of the disease. They do not cure it. The medicines must be taken at precise times. They have many unpleasant side effects. For some people, the medications work less well than for others. Other aspects of HIV treatment are relief of symptoms and prevention and treatment of infection. Always follow Standard Precautions at work to help prevent the spread of HIV/AIDS.

Guidelines
HIV/AIDS

- Involuntary weight loss occurs in almost all people who develop AIDS. High-protein and high-calorie meals can help maintain a healthy weight.

- People with poor immune systems are more sensitive to infections. Wash your hands often. Keep everything clean.

- Residents who have infections of the mouth may need food that is low in acid and neither cold nor hot. Spicy seasonings should be removed. Soft or pureed foods may be easier to swallow. Liquid meals and fortified drinks may help ease the pain of chewing. Warm salt water or other rinses may ease sores of the mouth. Good mouth care is vital.

- A person who has nausea or vomiting should eat small frequent meals, if possible. The person should eat slowly. Encourage fluids in between meals. These residents must maintain intake of fluids to balance lost fluids.

- Residents with mild diarrhea may need frequent small meals that are low in fat, fiber, and milk products. If diarrhea is severe, the doctor may order a "BRAT" diet (a diet of bananas, rice, apples, and toast). This is helpful for short-term use.

- Numbness, tingling, and pain in the feet and legs is usually treated with medications. Going barefoot or wearing loose, soft slippers may be helpful. If blankets cause pain, a bed cradle can keep sheets and blankets from resting on legs and feet (Fig. 8-31).

- Residents with HIV/AIDS may have anxiety and depression. They often suffer the judgments of family, friends, and society. Some people blame them for their illness. People with HIV/AIDS may have tremendous stress. They may feel uncertainty about their illness, health care, and finances. They may also have lost people in their social support network of friends and family.

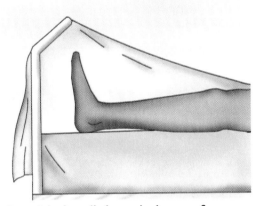

Fig. 8-31. **A bed cradle keeps bed covers from pushing down on a resident's feet.**

- Residents with HIV/AIDS need support from others. This may come from family, friends, religious and community groups, and support groups, as well as the healthcare team. Treat all your residents with respect. Help give the emotional support they need.

- Withdrawal, avoidance of tasks, and mental slowness are early symptoms of HIV infection. Medications may also cause side effects of this type. AIDS dementia complex may cause further mental symptoms. There may also be muscle weakness and loss of muscle control, making falls a risk. Residents will need a safe environment and close supervision in their ADLs.

Cancer

Cancer is a general term used to describe many types of malignant tumors. A **tumor** is a cluster of abnormally growing cells. Benign tumors grow slowly in local areas. They are considered non-cancerous. Malignant tumors grow rapidly. They invade surrounding tissues.

Cancer invades local tissue. It can spread to other parts of the body. Cancer can spread from the site where it first appeared and affect other body systems. In general, treatment is harder and cancer is more deadly after this has occurred. Cancer often appears first in the breast, colon, rectum, uterus, prostate, lungs, or skin.

Risk factors that appear to contribute to cancer are:

- tobacco use

- exposure to sunlight

- excessive alcohol intake

- exposure to some chemicals and industrial agents

- some food additives

- radiation

- poor nutrition

- lack of physical activity

When diagnosed early, cancer can often be treated and controlled. The American Cancer Society has identified seven warning signs of cancer:

1. **C**hange in bowel or bladder habits

2. **A** sore that does not heal

3. **U**nusual bleeding or discharge

4. **T**hickening or lump in the breast or elsewhere

5. **I**ndigestion or difficulty swallowing

6. **O**bvious change in a wart or mole

7. **N**agging cough or persistent hoarseness

People with cancer may live longer and can sometimes recover if they are treated early. Treatments include:

- surgery

- chemotherapy

- radiation (Fig. 8-32)

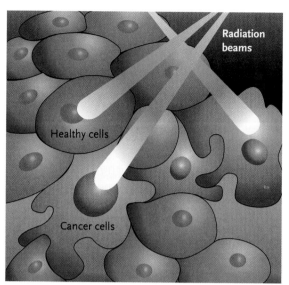

Fig. 8-32. Radiation is targeted at cancer cells, but it also destroys some healthy cells in its path.

Guidelines
Cancer

- **Each case is different**. Cancer is a general term. It refers to many separate situations. Residents may live many years or only several months. Treatment affects each person differently. Do not make assumptions about a resident's condition.

- **Communication**. Residents may want to talk or may avoid talking. Respect their needs. Be honest. Never say, "everything will be okay." Be sensitive. Remember that cancer is a disease. Its cause is unknown. Have a good attitude.

- **Nutrition**. Good nutrition is important for residents with cancer. Follow the care plan carefully. Use plastic utensils for a resident receiving chemotherapy. It makes food taste better. Silver utensils cause a bitter taste. Residents often have poor appetites. Encourage a variety of food and small portions.

- **Pain control**. Cancer can cause terrible pain, especially in the late stages. Watch for signs of pain. Report them to the nurse. Help with comfort measures, such as repositioning and providing conversation, music, or reading materials.

- **Comfort.** Give back rubs for comfort and to increase circulation. For residents who spend many hours in bed, sheepskins may be more comfortable. Moving to a chair may improve comfort as well. Residents who are weak or immobile need to be repositioned every two hours.

- **Skin care**. Use lotion on dry or delicate skin. Do not apply lotion to areas receiving radiation therapy. Do not remove markings that are used in radiation therapy. Follow any special skin care orders (for example: no hot or cold packs, no soap or cosmetics, no tight stockings).

- **Oral care**. Help residents brush and floss teeth regularly. Medications, nausea, vomiting, or mouth infections may cause a bad taste in the mouth. You can help by using a soft-bristled toothbrush, rinsing with baking soda and water, or using a prescribed rinse. Do not use a commercial mouthwash.

- **Self-image**. People with cancer may have a low self-image because they are weak and their appearance has changed. For example, hair loss is a common side effect of chemotherapy. Be sensitive. Help with grooming if it is desired.

- **Psychosocial needs**. If visitors help cheer your resident, encourage them. Do not intrude. If some times of day are better than others, suggest this. It may help a person with cancer to think of something else for a while. Pursue other topics. Get to know what interests your residents have.

- **Family assistance**. Having a family member with cancer can be very difficult. Be alert to needs that are not being met or stresses created by the illness.

Many services and support groups exist for people with cancer and their families or caregivers. Hospitals, hospice programs, and religious organizations have many resources. These include meal services, transportation to doctors' offices, counseling, and support groups. Check the yellow pages under "cancer," or call the American Cancer Society.

Unit 10. Describe mental illness, depression and related care

You first learned about mental health and mental illness in chapter 2. You can review the communication guidelines for mentally ill residents in that chapter.

There are many degrees of mental illness. It ranges from mild to severe.

Depression. Clinical depression is a serious mental illness. It may cause intense mental, emotional, and physical pain, and disability. It makes other illnesses worse. If untreated, it may result in suicide.

Sadness is only one symtpom of this illness (Fig. 8-33).

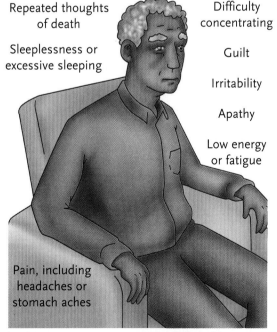

Repeated thoughts of death

Sleeplessness or excessive sleeping

Difficulty concentrating

Guilt

Irritability

Apathy

Low energy or fatigue

Pain, including headaches or stomach aches

Fig. 8-33. Common symptoms of clinical depression.

Other common symptoms of clinical depression include:

- pain, including headaches, stomach pain, and other body aches

- low energy or fatigue

- **apathy**, or lack of interest

- irritability

- anxiety

- loss of appetite

- problems with sexual functioning and desire

- sleeplessness, trouble sleeping, or excessive sleeping

- guilt

- trouble concentrating

- frequent thoughts of suicide and death

There are different types and degrees of depression. Major depression may cause a person to lose interest in everything he once cared about. Manic depression, or bipolar disorder, causes a person to swing from deep depression to extreme activity. These episodes include high energy, little sleep, big speeches, rapidly changing moods, high self-esteem, overspending, and poor judgment.

People cannot overcome depression through sheer will. It is an illness like any other illness. It can be treated successfully. People who suffer from depression need compassion and support. Know the symptoms. Recognize the beginning or worsening of depression. Any suicide threat should be taken seriously. Report it immediately. It should not be regarded as an attempt to get attention.

Anxiety-related Disorders. Anxiety is uneasiness or fear, often about a situation or condition. When a mentally healthy person feels anxiety, he or she usually knows the cause. The anxiety fades once the cause is removed. A mentally ill person may feel anxiety all the time. He or she may not know the reason why. Physical signs of anxiety-related disorders include shakiness, muscle aches, sweating, cold and clammy hands, dizziness, fatigue, racing heart, cold or hot flashes, a choking or smothering sensation, or a dry mouth.

Phobias are an intense form of anxiety. Many people are very afraid of some things or situations. Examples are fear of dogs or of flying. For a mentally ill person, a phobia is a disabling terror. It keeps the person from doing normal things. For example, the fear of being in a confined space, claustrophobia, may make using an elevator a terrifying task. Other anxiety-related disorders include **panic disorder**, in which a person is terrified for no known reason. **Obsessive compulsive disorder** is obsessive behavior a person uses to cope with anxiety. For example, a person may wash his hands over and over as a way of dealing with anxiety. Anxiety-related disorders may also be caused by a traumatic experience. This is known as **post-traumatic stress disorder**.

Guidelines
Mentally Ill Residents

- Observe residents carefully for changes in condition or abilities. Document and report your observations.

- Support the resident and his family and friends. Your positive, professional attitude encourages them.

- Encourage residents to do as much for themselves as possible. Be patient, supportive, and positive.

- Mental illness can be treated. Medication and psychotherapy are common methods. Drugs must be taken properly to promote benefits and reduce side effects.

Observing and Reporting Mentally Ill Residents

- changes in ability

- positive or negative mood changes, especially withdrawal (Fig. 8-34)

- behavior changes, including changes in personality, extreme behavior, and behavior that does not seem to fit the situation

- comments, even jokes, about hurting self or others

- failure to take medicine or improper use of medicine

- real or imagined physical symptoms

- events, situations, or people that seem to upset or excite residents

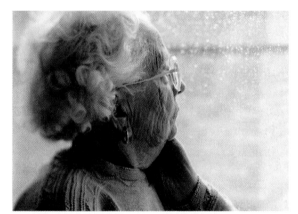

Fig. 8-34. **Withdrawal is an important change to report.**

nine
Rehabilitation and Restorative Services

Unit 1. Discuss rehabilitation and restorative care

When a resident loses some ability to function due to illness or injury, rehabilitation may be ordered. **Rehabilitation** is managed by professionals. It helps to restore a person to the highest possible level of functioning. These professionals include physical, occupational, and speech therapists.

Rehabilitation involves all parts of the person's disability. This includes psychological effects. The therapy used and the progress made are based on:

- the type of illness or injury and how serious it is
- the person's overall health
- motivation of the resident and the rehabilitation team
- when rehabilitation began

Goals of rehabilitation include:

- helping a resident regain function or recover from illness
- developing a resident's independence
- helping a resident control his or her life
- helping a resident adapt to the limitations of a disability

Restorative services usually follow rehabilitation. The goal is to keep the resident at the level achieved by rehabilitation. Restorative services also take a team approach. Staff create a care plan that includes the goals of restorative care. You will be an important member of this team. Nursing assistants spend more time with the residents than other team members. You play a critical role in recovery and independence. Along with required tasks, remember to:

- Be patient.
- Be positive and supportive.
- Focus only on small tasks and small accomplishments.
- Recognize that setbacks occur.
- Be sensitive to the resident's needs.
- Encourage independence.

RA *No matter what loss of function a resident has suffered, he or she has the right to expect staff to respond to his or her needs professionally—without judgment or bias.*

Observing and Reporting
Restorative Care

- any increase or decrease in abilities
- any change in attitude or motivation, positive or negative

- any change in general health, such as changes in skin condition, appetite, energy level, or general appearance

- signs of depression or mood changes

Unit 2. Describe the importance of promoting independence and list ways exercise improves health

Maintaining independence is vital during and after rehabilitation and restorative services. When an active and independent person becomes dependent, physical and mental problems may result. The body becomes less mobile. The mind is less focused. Studies show that the more active a person is, the better the mind and body work.

The staff's job is to keep residents as active as possible—physically and mentally. **Ambulation** is walking. A resident who is ambulatory can get out of bed and walk. Residents should ambulate to maintain independence and prevent problems. Lack of mobility may cause a loss of:

- independence
- self-esteem
- ability to move without help
- muscle strength, leading to contractures
- circulation of blood

Regular ambulation and exercise help improve:

- quality and health of the skin
- circulation
- strength
- sleep and relaxation
- appetite
- elimination
- blood flow
- oxygen level

Promoting social interaction and thinking abilities is important too. Most facilities have activities geared to residents' ages and abilities. Social involvement should be encouraged. When possible, nursing assistants should join in activities with residents. This promotes independence. It also gives nursing assistants a chance to observe residents' abilities.

📄 *The annual survey will look at the activities offered in the facility and see if all residents have an equal opportunity to participate.*

Unit 3. Describe assistive devices and equipment

Many devices help people who are recovering from or adapting to a physical condition. This equipment is called **assistive** or **adaptive devices**. Examples are shown below in Figure 9-1.

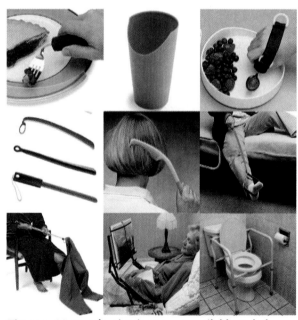

Fig. 9-1. Many adaptive items are available to help make it easier for residents to adapt to physical changes. (Photos courtesy of North Coast Medical, Inc., www.ncmedical.com, 800-821-9319)

- Adaptive equipment helps residents do ADLs. Each adaptive device is made to support a particular disability.

- Personal care equipment includes long-handled brushes and combs.

- Supportive devices are used when ambulating. Canes, walkers and crutches are examples.

- Safety devices, such as shower chairs and gait or transfer belts (Fig. 9-2), prevent accidents.

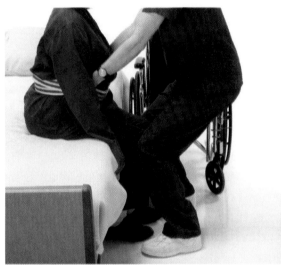

Fig. 9-2. A transfer belt, or gait belt, is used to assist residents who are able to walk but are weak or unsteady. The belt is made of canvas or other heavy material.

Check the care plan before helping a resident ambulate. Discuss the resident's abilities and disabilities with the nurse. Know the resident's limitations. Know the goals for restoring and maintaining function. Any time you help a resident, communicate what you would like to do. Let him do what he can do. The two of you will have to work together, especially during transfers.

When helping a visually-impaired resident walk, let the person walk beside and slightly behind you, as he rests a hand on your elbow. Walk at a normal pace. Let the person know when you are about to turn a corner, or when a step is approaching. Tell him whether you will be stepping up or down.

Assisting a resident to ambulate

Equipment: transfer belt, non-skid shoes for the resident

1. **Wash hands.**
   Provides for infection control.

2. **Identify yourself by name. Identify the resident by name.**
   Resident has right to know identity of his or her caregiver. Addressing resident by name shows respect and establishes correct identification.

3. **Explain procedure to resident. Speak clearly, slowly, and directly. Maintain face-to-face contact whenever possible.**
   Promotes understanding and independence.

4. **Provide for resident's privacy with curtain, screen, or door.**
   Maintains resident's right to privacy and dignity.

5. **Before ambulating, put on and properly fasten non-skid footwear on resident.**
   Promotes resident's safety. Prevents falls.

6. **Adjust bed to a low position so that the feet are flat on the floor. Lock bed wheels.**
   Prevents injury and promotes stability.

7. **Stand in front of and face resident.**

8. **Brace resident's lower extremities. Bend your knees. If resident has a weak knee, brace it against your knee.**
   Promotes proper body mechanics. Reduces risk of back injury.

9. **With transfer (gait) belt: Place belt around resident's waist. Grasp the belt while assisting resident to stand.**

   Without transfer belt: Place arms around resident's torso under resident's armpits, while assisting resident to stand.

10. **With transfer belt: Walk slightly behind and to one side of resident for the full distance, while holding onto the transfer belt (Fig. 9-3).**

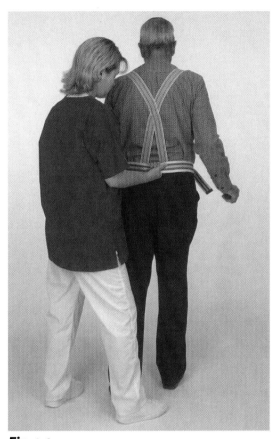

Fig. 9-3.

Without transfer belt: Walk slightly behind and to one side of resident for the full distance. Support resident's back with your arm.

11. **After ambulation, remove transfer belt if used. Help the resident to a position of comfort and safety.**

12. **Return bed to appropriate position. Remove privacy measures.**

13. **Before leaving, place call light within resident's reach.**
    Allows resident to communicate with staff as necessary.

14. **Wash hands.**
    Provides for infection control.

15. **Report any changes in resident to nurse.**
    Provides nurse with information to assess resident.

16. **Document procedure using facility guidelines.**
    What you write is a legal record of what you did. If you don't document it, legally it didn't happen.

👁 *Before assisting with ambulation, you must apply non-skid footwear to the resident. It reduces the risk of the resident slipping and/or falling.*

Residents who have trouble walking may use canes, walkers, or crutches to help themselves. A cane helps with balance. A straight cane is not designed to bear weight. A quad cane, with four rubber-tipped feet, is designed to bear a little weight (Fig. 9-4). Residents using canes should be able to bear weight on both legs. If one leg is weaker, the cane should be held in the hand on the strong side.

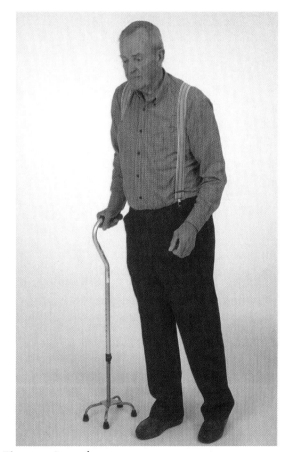

Fig. 9-4. A quad cane.

A walker is used when the resident can bear some weight on the legs. The walker gives stability for residents who are unsteady or lack balance. The metal frame may have rubber-tipped feet and/or wheels.

9

Rehabilitation and Restorative Services

Crutches are used for residents who can bear no weight or limited weight on one leg. Some people use one crutch. Some use two. Your role is to ensure safety. Stay near the resident. Stay on the weak side. Make sure the crutches are in good condition. They must be sturdy. They must have rubber tips on the bottom.

When a resident uses a walker or cane, follow these guidelines. They will help keep the resident safe.

Guidelines
Cane or Walker Use

- Be sure the resident is wearing non-skid shoes.

- Be sure the walker or cane is in good condition. It must have rubber tips on bottom. Walker may have wheels. If so, check the walker's wheels for safety.

- Have the resident use both hands on the walker. The walker should not be over-extended. It should be placed no more than 12 inches in front of the resident.

- Purses or clothing cannot hang on the walker.

- Have the resident use the cane on his or her strong side.

- Stay near the person, on the weak side.

- If height of the cane or walker does not fit a resident, tell the nurse or physical therapist.

Assisting with ambulation for a resident using a cane, walker, or crutches

Equipment: transfer belt, non-skid shoes for resident, cane, walker, or crutches

1. **Wash hands.**
   Provides for infection control.

2. **Identify yourself by name. Identify the resident by name.**
   Resident has right to know identity of his or her caregiver. Addressing resident by name shows respect and establishes correct identification.

3. **Explain procedure to resident. Speak clearly, slowly, and directly. Maintain face-to-face contact whenever possible.**
   Promotes understanding and independence.

4. **Provide for resident's privacy with curtain, screen, or door.**
   Maintains resident's right to privacy and dignity.

5. **Before ambulating, put on and properly fasten non-skid footwear on resident.**
   Promotes resident's safety. Prevents falls.

6. **Adjust bed to a low position so that the feet are flat on the floor. Lock bed wheels.**
   Prevents injury and promotes stability.

7. **Stand in front of and face resident.**

8. **Brace resident's lower extremities. Bend your knees. If resident has a weak knee, brace it against your knee.**
   Promotes proper body mechanics. Reduces risk of back injury.

9. **Place transfer belt around resident's waist and grasp the belt, while helping resident to stand.**
   Promotes resident's safety.

10. **Help as needed with ambulation.**

a. *Cane.* **Resident places cane about 12 inches in front of his stronger leg. He brings weaker leg even with cane. He then brings stronger leg forward slightly ahead of cane. Repeat (Fig. 9-5).**

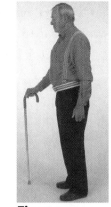

Fig. 9-5.

b. *Walker.* **Resident picks up or rolls the walker. He places it about 12 inches in front of him. All four feet or wheels of the walker should be on the ground before resident steps forward to the walker. The walker should not be** moved again until the resident has moved both feet forward and is steady (Fig. 9-6). The resident should never put his feet ahead of the walker.

Promotes stability and prevents falls.

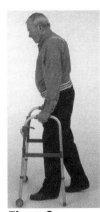

Fig. 9-6.

c. **Crutches.** Resident should be fitted for crutches and taught to use them correctly by a physical therapist or nurse. The resident may use the crutches several different ways. It depends on what his weakness is. No matter how they are used, weight should be on the resident's hands and arms. Weight should not be on the underarm area (Fig. 9-7).

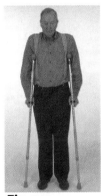

Fig. 9-7.

11. Walk slightly behind and to one side of resident. Hold the transfer belt if one is used.

Provides security.

12. Watch for obstacles in the resident's path. Ask the resident to look ahead, not down down at his feet.

Promotes resident's safety. Prevents injury.

13. Encourage resident to rest if he is tired. When a resident is tired, it increases the chance of a fall. Let resident set the pace. Discuss how far he plans to go based on the care plan.

Prevents falls.

14. After ambulation, remove transfer belt. Help resident to a position of comfort and safety.

15. Return bed to appropriate position. Remove privacy measures.

16. Before leaving, place call light within resident's reach.

Allows resident to communicate with staff as necessary.

17. Wash hands.

Provides for infection control.

18. Report any changes in resident to nurse.

Provides nurse with information to assess resident.

19. Document procedure using facility guidelines.

What you write is a legal record of what you did. If you don't document it, legally it didn't happen.

👁 *You will be expected to promote residents' safety in all procedures you demonstrate.*

Unit 4. Describe positioning and how to assist with range of motion (ROM) exercises

Residents who spend a lot of time in bed often need help getting into comfortable positions. They also need to change positions periodically. This helps avoid muscle stiffness and skin breakdown or pressure sores.

Positioning means helping residents into positions that will be comfortable and healthy for them. Bedbound residents should be repositioned every two hours. Document the position and time every time there is a change.

Following are the five basic body positions:

1. **Supine** or lying flat on back (Fig. 9-8)

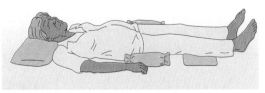

Fig. 9-8. A person in the supine position is lying flat on her back.

9

Rehabilitation and Restorative Services

2. **Lateral** or side (Fig. 9-9)

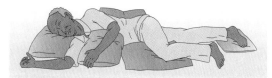

Fig. 9-9. A person in the lateral position is lying on his side.

3. **Prone** or lying on the stomach (Fig. 9-10)

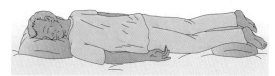

Fig. 9-10. A person in the prone position is lying on his stomach.

4. **Fowler's** or partially reclined (Fig. 9-11)

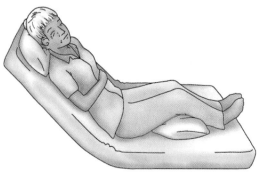

Fig. 9-11. A person lying in the Fowler's position is partially reclined.

5. **Sims'** or lying on the left side with one leg drawn up (Fig. 9-12)

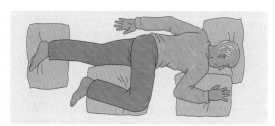

Fig. 9-12. A person lying in the Sims' position is lying on his left side with one leg drawn up.

Residents who are confined to bed need good body alignment. This aids recovery and prevents injury to muscles and joints. These guidelines help residents maintain good alignment and make progress when they can get out of bed.

Guidelines
Alignment and Positioning

- Observe principles of alignment. Proper alignment is based on straight lines. The spine should be in a straight line. Pillows or rolled or folded blankets can support the small of the back and raise the knees or head in the supine position. They can support the head and one leg in the lateral position.

- Keep body parts in natural positions. In a natural hand position, the fingers are slightly curled. Use a rolled washcloth, gauze bandage, or a rubber ball inside the palm to support the fingers in this position (Fig. 9-13). Use bed cradles to keep covers from resting on feet in the supine position. Footboards are padded boards placed against the resident's feet to keep them flexed (chapter 5).

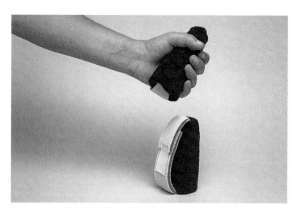

Fig. 9-13. Handrolls keep fingers from curling tightly. (Reprinted with permission of the Briggs Corporation, 800-247-2343)

- Prevent external rotation of hips. When legs and hips turn outward during bedrest, hip contractures can result. A trochanter roll, or a rolled blanket or towel tucked alongside the hip and thigh can keep the leg from turning outward (see Fig. 9-8).

- Change positions often to prevent muscle stiffness and pressure sores. This should be done at least every two hours. The positions used will depend on the resident's condition and preference. Check the skin every time you reposition the resident.

• Have plenty of pillows available to provide support in the various positions.

• Use positioning devices (backrests, bed cradles, draw sheets, footboards, and hand rolls). Splints may be prescribed by a doctor to keep a resident's joints in the correct position (Fig. 9-14).

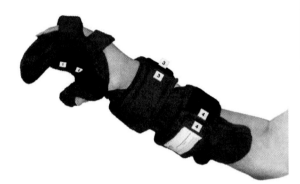

Fig. 9-14. One type of splint. (Photo courtesy of Lenjoy Medical Engineering "Comfy Splints™" 800-582-5332, www.comfysplints.com)

• Give back rubs as ordered for comfort and relaxation.

Exercise helps people regain strength and mobility. It helps to prevent disabilities. People who are in bed for long periods are more likely to develop contractures. **Contractures** are the permanent and often painful stiffening of a joint and muscle. They are often caused by immobility. They can result in the loss of ability.

Range of motion (ROM) exercises put a joint through its full arc of motion. The goal of range of motion exercises is to decrease or prevent contractures, improve strength, and increase circulation. Passive range of motion (PROM) exercises are used when residents cannot move on their own. When helping with PROM exercises, support the resident's joints. Move them through the range of motion. Active range of motion

(AROM) exercises are done by a resident himself. Your role in AROM exercises is to encourage the resident. Active assisted range of motion (AAROM) exercises are done by the resident with some help and support from you.

You will not do ROM exercises without an order from a doctor, nurse, or physical therapist. Follow the care plan. You will repeat each exercise three to five times, once or twice a day. You will work on both sides of the body. During ROM exercises, begin at the resident's head. Work down the body. Exercise the upper extremities (arms) before the lower extremities (legs). Give support above and below the joint.

Stop the motion if the resident reports pain. Report pain to the nurse. These exercises are specific for each body area. They include these movements (Fig. 9-15):

• **Abduction**: moving a body part away from the body

• **Adduction**: moving a body part toward the body

• **Dorsiflexion**: bending backward

• **Rotation**: turning a joint

• **Extension**: straightening a body part

• **Flexion**: bending a body part

• **Pronation**: turning downward

• **Supination**: turning upward

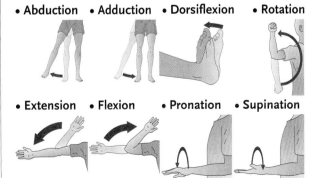

Fig. 9-15.

Assisting with passive range of motion exercises

1. **Wash hands.**

   Provides for infection control.

2. **Identify yourself by name. Identify the resident by name.**

   Resident has right to know identity of his or her caregiver. Addressing resident by name shows respect and establishes correct identification.

3. **Explain procedure to resident. Speak clearly, slowly, and directly. Maintain face-to-face contact whenever possible.**

   Promotes understanding and independence.

4. **Provide for resident's privacy with curtain, screen, or door.**

   Maintains resident's right to privacy and dignity.

5. **Adjust bed to a safe working level, usually waist high. Lock bed wheels.**

   Prevents injury to you and to resident.

6. **Position the resident lying supine—flat on his or her back—on the bed. Position body in good alignment.**

   Reduces stress to joints.

7. **Repeat each exercise at least 3 times.**

8. ***Shoulder.* Support resident's arm at elbow and wrist while performing ROM for shoulder. Place one hand under the elbow and the other hand under the wrist. Raise the straightened arm from the side position forward to above the head and return arm to side of the body (flexion/extension) (Fig. 9-16).**

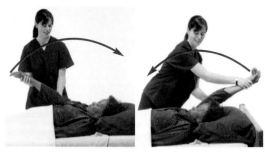

Fig. 9-16.

Raise the arm to side position above head and return arm to side of the body.

(abduction/adduction) (Fig. 9-17).

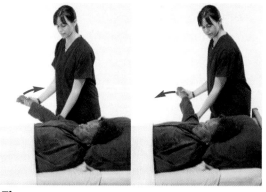

Fig. 9-17.

9. ***Elbow.* Hold the wrist with one hand. Hold the elbow with the other hand. Bend elbow so that the hand touches the shoulder on that same side (flexion). Straighten arm (extension) (Fig. 9-18).**

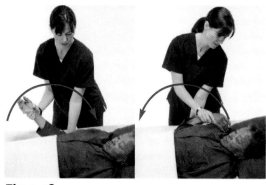

Fig. 9-18.

Exercise forearm by moving it so palm is facing downward (pronation) and then upward (supination) (Fig. 9-19).

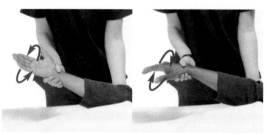

Fig. 9-19.

10. ***Wrist.* Hold the wrist with one hand. Use the fingers of the other hand to help the joint through the motions. Bend the hand down (flexion). Bend the hand backwards (extension) (Fig. 9-20).**

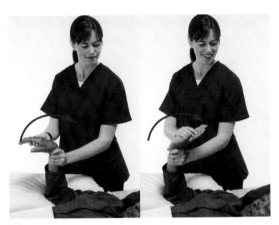

Fig. 9-20.

Turn the hand in the direction of the thumb (radial flexion). Then turn the hand in the direction of the little finger (ulnar flexion) (Fig. 9-21).

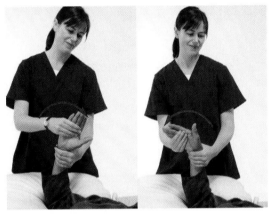

Fig. 9-21.

11. *Thumb.* Move the thumb away from the index finger (abduction). Move the thumb back next to the index finger (adduction) (Fig. 9-22).

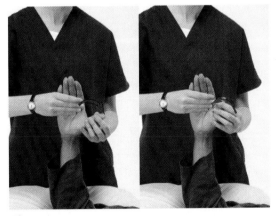

Fig. 9-22.

Touch each fingertip with the thumb (opposition) (Fig. 9-23).

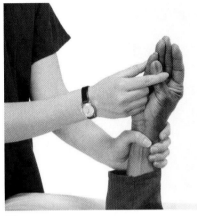

Fig. 9-23.

Bend thumb into the palm (flexion) and out to the side (extension) (Fig. 9-24).

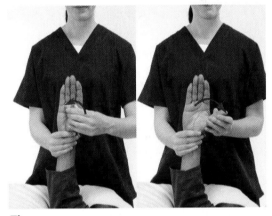

Fig. 9-24.

12. *Fingers.* Make the hand into a fist (flexion). Gently straighten out the fist (extension) (Fig. 9-25).

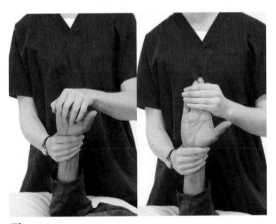

Fig. 9-25.

Spread the fingers and the thumb far apart from each other (abduction). Bring the fingers back next to each other (adduction) (Fig. 9-26).

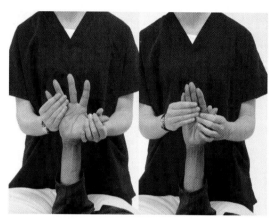

Fig. 9-26.

13. *Hip.* Support the leg by placing one hand under the knee and one under the ankle. Straighten the leg. Raise it gently upward. Move the leg away from the other leg (abduction). Move the leg toward the other leg (adduction) (Fig. 9-27).

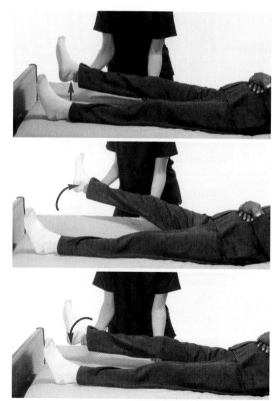

Fig. 9-27.

Gently turn the leg inward (internal rotation). Turn the leg outward (external rotation) (Fig. 9-28).

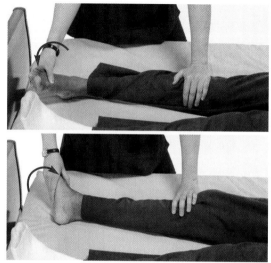

Fig. 9-28.

14. *Knees.* Support resident's leg under the knee and ankle while performing ROM for knee. Bend the knee to the point of resistance (flexion). Return leg to resident's normal position. (extension) (Fig. 9-29).

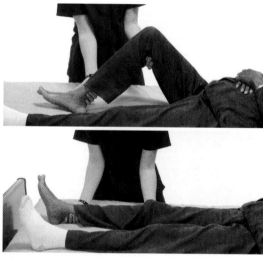

Fig. 9-29.

15. *Ankles.* Support the foot and ankle close to the bed while performing ROM for the ankle. Push/pull foot up toward head (dorsiflexion). Push/pull foot down, with the toes pointed down (plantar flexion) (Fig. 9-30).

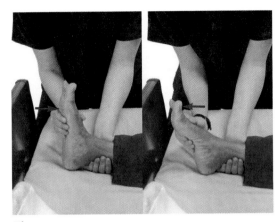

Fig. 9-30.

Turn inside of the foot inward toward the body (supination). Bend the sole of the foot away from the body (pronation) (Fig. 9-31).

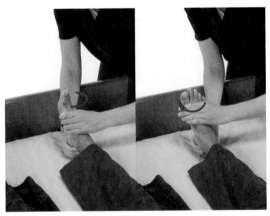

Fig. 9-31.

16. *Toes.* Curl and straighten the toes (flexion and extension) (Fig. 9-32).

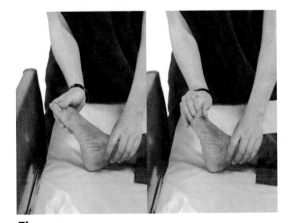

Fig. 9-32.

Gently spread the toes apart (abduction) (Fig. 9-33).

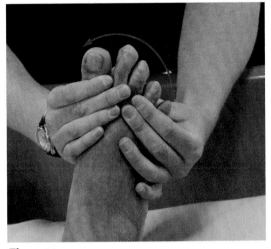

Fig. 9-33.

17. **While supporting the limbs, move all joints gently, slowly, and smoothly through the range of motion to the point of resistance. Stop exercises if any pain occurs.**
    Rapid movement may cause injury. Pain is a warning sign for injury.

18. **Return bed to proper position. Remove privacy measures.**
    Promotes resident's safety.

19. **Before leaving, place call light within resident's reach.**
    Allows resident to communicate with staff as necessary.

20. **Wash hands.**
    Provides for infection control.

21. **Report any changes in resident to nurse.**
    Provides nurse with information to assess resident.

22. **Document procedure using facility guidelines.**
    What you write is a legal record of what you did. If you don't document it, legally it didn't happen.

👁 *When taking the certification exam, you may not be tested on ROM exercises for the entire body. You may only be tested on specific body parts. Regardless, it is important to remember that during ROM exercises, you must support the limbs at all times. Move joints gently and slowly. Always stop if pain occurs. Pain is a warning sign for injury.*

9

Rehabilitation and Restorative Services

Unit 5. List guidelines for assisting with bowel and bladder retraining

Injury, illness, or inactivity may cause a loss of normal bowel or bladder function. Residents may need help to re-establish a regular bathroom routine. Problems with elimination can be embarrassing or difficult to talk about. Be sensitive.

Residents may have incontinence. **Incontinence** is the inability to control the bowels or bladder (Fig. 9-34). Always be professional when handling incontinence or helping to re-establish routines. Never show anger or frustration toward residents who are incontinent. The problem is out of their control. Be positive. Never refer to an incontinence brief or pad as a "diaper." Residents are not children. This is disrespectful.

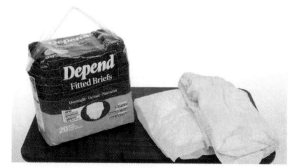

Fig. 9-34. A type of incontinence pad.

Guidelines
Bowel or Bladder Retraining

- Follow Standard Precautions. Wear gloves when handling body wastes.

- Explain the training schedule to the resident. Follow the schedule carefully.

- Keep a record of the residents' bowel and bladder habits. When you see a pattern of elimination, you can predict when the resident will need a bedpan or a trip to the bathroom.

- Offer a commode or a trip to the bathroom before beginning long procedures (Fig. 9-35).

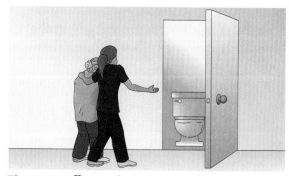

Fig. 9-35. Offer regular trips to the bathroom.

- Encourage residents to drink plenty of fluids. Do this even if urinary incontinence is a problem. About 30 minutes after fluids are taken, offer a trip to the bathroom or a bedpan or urinal.

- Encourage the resident to eat foods that are high in fiber, as allowed.

- Answer call lights promptly. Residents cannot wait long when the urge to go to the bathroom occurs. Leave call lights within reach (Fig. 9-36).

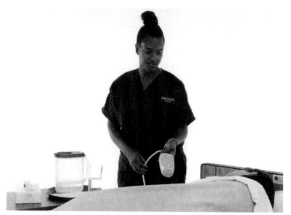

Fig. 9-36. Leave call lights within reach. Answer call lights promptly.

- Provide privacy for elimination—both in the bed and in the bathroom.

- If the resident has difficulty urinating, try running the water in the sink. Have him or her lean forward slightly. This puts pressure on the bladder.

- Do not rush the resident.

- Help residents with good perineal care. This prevents skin breakdown and promotes proper hygiene. Carefully observe for skin changes.

- Discard wastes according to facility rules.

- Discard clothing protectors and incontinence briefs properly. Some facilities require double-bagging these items. This stops odors from collecting.

- Some facilities use washable bed pads or briefs. Follow Standard Precautions when rinsing before placing these items in the laundry.

- Keep an accurate record of urination and bowel movements. This includes episodes of incontinence.

- Praise successes, or attempts, to control bowel and bladder.

When the resident is incontinent or cannot toilet when asked, be positive. Never make the resident feel like a failure. Praise and encouragement are essential for a successful program. Some residents will always be incontinent. Be patient. Offer these persons extra care and attention. Skin breakdown may lead to pressure sores without proper care. Always report changes in skin.

RA *Be professional when handling incontinence. It is hard enough for residents to handle incontinence without having to worry about your reactions. Showing frustration or anger is abusive behavior. Negative reactions only make the problem worse. Be patient when setbacks occur.*

Unit 6. **Describe care and use of prosthetic devices**

Amputation is the removal of some or all of a body part. It is usually a foot, hand, arm or leg. Amputation may be the result of an injury or disease. After amputation, some people feel that the limb is still there. They may feel pain in the part that has been amputated. This is called **phantom sensation**. It may last for a short time or for years. The pain or sensation is caused by remaining nerve endings. It is real. It should not be ignored or made fun of.

A **prosthesis** is an artificial body part. It replaces a missing body part, such as an eye, arm, hand, foot, or leg. The prosthesis will be custom-fitted to the resident (Fig. 9-37). When a body part has been amputated, day-to-day activities may be limited. A resident will need special care to help him adjust to these changes. When the condition is new and a prosthesis has been ordered, a physical and/or occupational therapist may work with the resident.

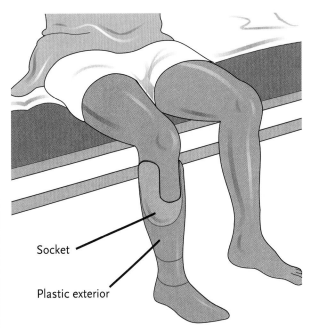

Socket

Plastic exterior

Fig. 9-37. **Prostheses are specially-fitted, expensive pieces of equipment.**

You will help with ADLs and ambulation. You must know how to care for the limb and how to use a prosthesis. Prostheses are expensive. Take great care with them.

Guidelines
Amputation and Prosthesis Care

- Residents who have had a body part amputated must make many physical, psychological, social, and occupational adjustments to their disability. Be very supportive.

- Help residents with ADLs.

- Follow the care plan for care of the prosthesis and the limb.

- A nurse or therapist will demonstrate application of a prosthesis. Follow instructions to apply and remove the prosthesis. Follow the manufacturer's care directions.

- Keep a prosthesis and the skin under it dry and clean.

- If ordered, apply a stump sock before putting on the prosthesis.

- Observe the skin on stump. Watch for signs of skin breakdown caused by pressure and abrasion. Report any redness or open areas.

- Check with the nurse prior to exercising to see if pain medication is needed.

- Phantom sensation is real pain and should be treated that way.

- Never try to fix a prosthesis. Report any problems to the nurse.

- Do not show negative feelings about the stump during care.

- If the resident has an artificial eye, review the care plan with the nurse. Some artificial eyes will be surgically implanted into the eye socket. They will not be removed for cleaning. Others are removed for cleaning and storage. Artificial eyes are made of glass or plastic. They must be handled very carefully. Never clean or soak the eye in alcohol. It will crack the plastic and destroy it. If the prosthesis must be removed, store it in water or saline. The resident will usually be taught how to remove, clean, and insert the eye. Know any special instructions for assisting the resident with care.

- Again, take care when handling a prosthesis. They are very expensive (an artificial leg may cost from $10,000 to $20,000).

ten
Caring for Yourself

Unit 1. Describe how to find a job

If you are in school, you may soon be looking for a job. To find a job, you must first find potential employers. Then you must contact them to find out about job opportunities. To find employers, use the newspaper, the telephone book, the Internet, or personal contacts (Fig. 10-1). Ask your instructor about potential employers. Some schools keep a list of potential employers.

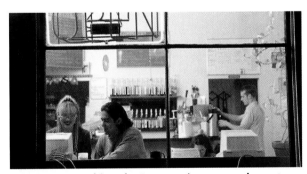

Fig. 10-1. **Searching the Internet is one good way to find a job.**

Once you have a good list of potential employers, you need to contact them. Phoning first is a good way to learn what jobs are available and how to apply.

When making an appointment, ask what information to bring with you. Make sure you have it when you go. Some documents you may need to show a potential employer are:

- Identification: driver's license, social security card, birth certificate, passport, or other official form of identification

- Proof of your legal status in this country and proof that you are legally able to work, even if you're a U.S.-born citizen. Employers must have files showing that employees are legally allowed to work in this country. Do not be upset by this request.

- High school diploma or equivalency, school transcripts, and diploma or certificate from your nursing assistant training course. It is a good idea to have your instructor's name and phone number, too.

- References are people who can be called to recommend you as an employee. They can include former employers, former teachers, or your minister. Do not use relatives or friends. You can ask them beforehand to write letters for you, addressed "To whom it may concern," explaining how they know you and describing your skills, qualities, and habits. Take copies of these with you.

On one sheet of paper, write down the general information you will need to complete an application. Take it with you. This will save time and avoid mistakes.

10

Caring for Yourself

Include the following general information:

- your address and phone number

- your birth date

- your social security number

- the name and address of the school or program where you were trained and the date you completed it, as well as certification numbers and expiration dates from a nursing assistant certification card, if you have one

- the names, titles, addresses, and phone numbers of former employers, and the dates you worked there

- salary information from your former jobs

- why you left each of your former jobs

- the names, addresses, and phone numbers of your references

- the days and hours you can work (facilities usually have shifts on days, nights, and weekends)

- a brief statement of why you are changing jobs or why you want to work as a nursing assistant

Fill out the application carefully and neatly (Fig. 10-2). Never lie. Before you write anything, read it all the way through. If you do not understand what is being asked, find out before filling in that space. Do not leave anything blank. You may write N/A (not applicable) if the question does not apply to you.

By law, your employer must do a criminal background check. You may be asked to sign a form granting permission to do this. Do not take it personally. It is a law intended to protect residents.

Use these tips to make the best impression at a job interview:

- Dress neatly and appropriately.

- Shower or bathe. Use deodorant.

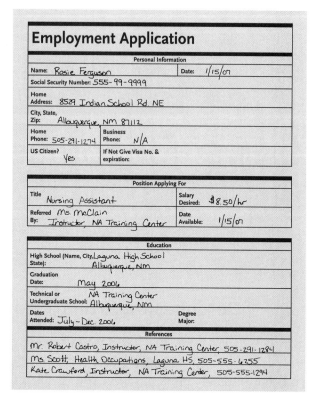

Fig. 10-2. A sample job application.

- Wash your hands. Clean and file your nails. Nails should be medium length or shorter.

- Men should shave right before the interview.

- Brush your teeth.

- Do not smoke. You will smell like smoke during the interview.

- Do not wear perfume or cologne. Many people dislike or are allergic to scents.

- Wear only simple makeup and jewelry or none at all.

- Wear your hair in a simple style.

- Wear a nice pair of pants, a skirt or a dress. Make sure your clothes are not wrinkled. A skirt or dress should be no shorter than knee-length. Do not wear jeans or shorts.

- Make sure your shoes are polished. Do not wear sneakers or open-toed sandals.

- Arrive 10 or 15 minutes early.

- Introduce yourself. Smile and shake

10

Caring for Yourself

hands (Fig. 10-3). Your handshake should be firm and confident.

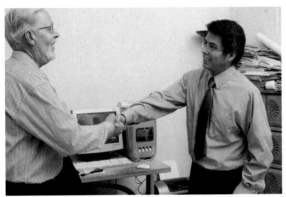

Fig. 10-3. Smile and shake hands confidently when you arrive at a job interview.

- Answer all questions clearly and completely.
- Make eye contact to show you are sincere (Fig. 10-4).
- Avoid using slang words or expressions.
- Never eat, drink, chew gum, or smoke in an interview.
- Sit up or stand up straight. Look happy to be there.
- Do not bring friends or children with you.
- Relax. You have worked hard to get this far. Be confident!

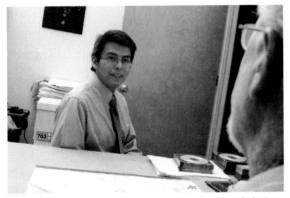

Fig. 10-4. Be polite and make eye contact while interviewing.

Be positive when answering questions. Emphasize what you enjoy or think you will enjoy about being a nursing assistant. Do not complain about previous jobs. Make it clear that you are hardworking and willing to work with all kinds of residents.

Usually interviewers will ask if you have any questions. Have some prepared. Write them down so you do not forget things you really want to know. Questions you may want to ask include:

- What hours would I work?
- What benefits does the job include? Is health insurance available? Would I get paid sick days or holidays?
- What orientation or training will be provided?
- Will my supervisor be available when needed?
- How soon will you be making a decision about this position?

Later in the interview, you may want to ask about salary or wages if you have not already been told what it would be. Listen carefully to the answers to your questions. Take notes if needed. You will probably be told when you can expect to hear from the employer. Do not expect to be offered a job at the interview. When the interview is over, stand up and shake hands again. Thank the employer for meeting with you.

Send a thank-you letter after every job interview. This states your continued interest in the position. If you have not heard back from the employer within the time frame you discussed with the interviewer, call and ask if the job was filled.

Unit 2. Describe ways to be a great employee

Handling criticism is hard for most people. Being able to accept and learn from criticism is important in all relationships, including employment. From time to time you will get

10

Caring for Yourself

evaluations from your employer. They contain ideas to help you improve your job performance. Here are some tips for handling criticism and using it to your benefit:

- Listen to the message that is being sent. Do not get so upset that you cannot understand the message.

- Hostile criticism and constructive criticism are not the same. Hostile criticism is angry and negative. Examples are, "You are useless!" or, "You are lazy and slow." Hostile criticism should not come from your employer or supervisor. You may hear hostile criticism from residents, family members, or others. The best response is something like, "I'm sorry you are so disappointed," and nothing more. Give the person a chance to calm down before trying to discuss their comments.

- Constructive criticism may come from your employer, supervisor, or others. Constructive criticism is meant to help you improve. Examples are, "You really need to be more accurate in your charting," or, "You are late too often. You'll have to make more of an effort to be on time." Listening to and acting on constructive criticism can help you be more successful in your job. Pay attention to it (Fig. 10-5).

- If you are not sure how to avoid a mistake you have made, always ask for suggestions. Avoiding mistakes will help you improve your performance.

- Apologize and move on. If you have made a mistake, apologize as needed. This may be to your supervisor, a resident, or others. Learn from the incident and put it behind you. Do not dwell on it or hold a grudge. Responding professionally to criticism is important for success in any job.

Evaluations will also cover overall knowledge, conflict resolution, and team effort.

Flexibility, friendliness, trustworthiness, and customer service are other things considered. Evaluations are often the basis for salary increases. A good evaluation can help you advance within the facility. Being open to criticism and suggestions for improvement will help you be more successful.

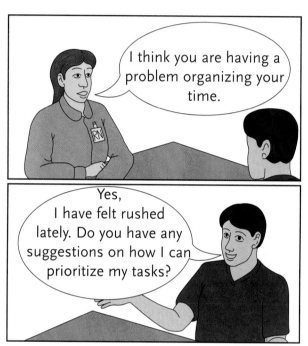

Fig. 10-5. Ask for suggestions when receiving constructive criticism.

If you decide to change jobs, be responsible. Always give your employer at least two weeks' written notice that you will be leaving. Otherwise, your facility may be understaffed. Both the residents and other staff will suffer. Future employers may talk with past supervisors. People who change jobs too often or who do not give notice before leaving are less likely to be hired.

Unit 3. Review guidelines for behaving professionally on the job

Be professional in your new job! This will help you keep your job. It will also help you earn the respect of co-workers and residents.

Remember the following:

- Be responsible; always call in if you cannot show up for a scheduled work shift.

- Be on time for your shift.

- Be clean and neatly dressed and groomed (Fig. 10-6).

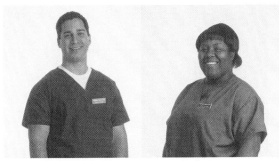

Fig. 10-6. Being clean and well-groomed is an important part of being a nursing assistant.

- Maintain a positive attitude.

- Follow policies and procedures.

- Document and report carefully and correctly.

- Ask questions when you do not know or understand something.

- Communicate with residents and members of the care team.

- Report anything that keeps you from completing duties.

- Offer positive suggestions for improving care.

Unit 4. Identify guidelines for maintaining certification and explain the state's registry

To meet OBRA's requirements, several organizations, including the National Council of State Boards of Nursing, created competency evaluation programs. These programs are a guide for each state for developing NA testing programs. OBRA requires that NAs complete at least 75 hours of training before being employed. Many states' requirements exceed the minimum 75 hours.

After completing a state's required hours of training, NAs may then take the test in that state. A fee may be charged. Once a nursing assistant has passed both the written and manual skills test, a certificate is mailed. Each state has different requirements for maintaining certification. Learn your state's requirements. Follow them exactly or you will not be able to keep working. Ask your instructor or employer for the requirements in your state. Know how long an absence from working as a nursing assistant is allowed without losing your certification.

Your employer may require that you show proof of renewal of your certificate each time it expires. Do not let your certificate expire. Respond immediately to your state's request to renew your certification. There may be a fee.

In the United States, each state keeps a registry for certified nursing assistants (CNAs). This registry keeps track of each nursing assistant working in that state. Information kept in the registry includes:

- a nursing assistant's full name and any other names the person may have used

- a nursing assistant's home address and other information, such as date of birth and social security number

- the date that a nursing assistant was placed in the registry and the results from the state test

- expiration dates of nursing assistants' certificates

- information about investigations and hearings regarding abuse, neglect, or theft, which becomes a part of a nursing assistant's permanent record

NAs can ask for a written statement to be added to the file. This includes information explaining events in the nursing assistants' own words. NAs have the right to correct any errors in a registry file.

Unit 5. Describe continuing education for nursing assistants

The federal government requires nursing assistants to have 12 hours of continuing education each year. Some states may require more. In-service continuing education courses help you keep your knowledge and skills fresh. Classes also give new information about conditions, challenges in working with residents, or regulation changes. Your facility must provide and document this continuing education. It is sometimes called an in-service.

Your employer is responsible for offering in-service courses. You are responsible for successfully attending and completing them. It is your responsibility to meet education requirements:

- Sign up for the course or find out where it is offered.

- Attend all class sessions.

- Pay attention and complete all the class requirements.

- Make the most of your in-service programs. Participate! (Fig. 10-7)

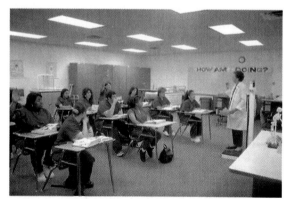

***Fig. 10-7.** Pay attention and participate during in-service courses.*

- Keep original copies of all certificates and

records of your successful attendance so you can prove you took the class.

📋 *The annual survey includes a review of personnel files to assure that all state and federal education, training, certification, and employee health regulations are met.*

Unit 6. Define "stress" and "stressors" and explain ways to manage stress

Stress is the state of being frightened, excited, confused, in danger, or irritated. We may think only bad things cause stress. However, positive situations cause stress, too. For example, getting married or having a baby are usually positive situations. But both can bring enormous stress from the changes they bring to our lives.

You may be thrilled when you get a new job as a nursing assistant. Starting work may also cause you stress. You may be afraid of making mistakes, excited about earning money or helping people, or confused about your new duties. Learning how to recognize stress and its causes is helpful. Then you can master a few simple methods for relaxing and learn to manage stress.

A **stressor** is something that causes stress. Anything can be a stressor. Some examples are:

- divorce

- marriage

- a new baby

- children leaving home

- feeling unprepared for a task

- starting a new job

- new responsibilities at work

- losing a job

- problems at work
- supervisors
- co-workers
- residents
- illness
- finances

Stress is not only an emotional response. It is also a physical response. When we have stress, changes occur in our bodies. The endocrine system may produce more of the hormone adrenaline. This can increase nervous system response, heart rate, respiratory rate, and blood pressure. This is why, in stressful situations, your heart beats fast, you breathe hard, and you feel warm or perspire.

Each of us has a different tolerance level for stress. What one person would find overwhelming may not bother another person. Your tolerance for stress depends on your personality, life experiences, and physical health.

Guidelines
Managing Stress

- Develop healthy habits of diet, exercise, and lifestyle.
- Eat nutritious foods.
- Exercise regularly (Fig. 10-8).

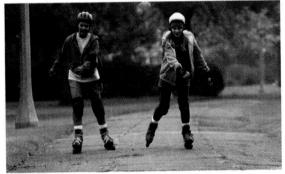

Fig. 10-8. Regular exercise is one healthy way to decrease stress.

- Get enough sleep.
- Drink only in moderation.
- Do not smoke.
- Find time at least a few times a week to do something relaxing, such as taking a walk, reading a book, or sewing.

Not managing stress can cause many problems. Some of these problems will affect how well you do your job. Signs that you are not managing stress are:

- showing anger or being abusive toward residents
- arguing with your supervisor about assignments
- having poor relationships with co-workers and residents
- complaining about your job and your responsibilities
- feeling work-related burn-out
- feeling tired even when you are rested
- trouble focusing on residents and procedures

RA *You may never hit a resident, **no matter what**. If you feel out of control, seek help, advice, or at least put some distance between you and the situation.*

Stress can seem overwhelming when you try to handle it yourself. Often just talking about stress or stressors can help you manage it better. Sometimes another person can offer helpful suggestions. You may think of new ways to handle stress just by talking it through. Get help from one or more of these when managing stress:

- your supervisor or another member of the care team for work-related stress
- your family
- your friends

10

Caring for Yourself

- your church, synagogue, mosque, or temple
- your doctor
- a local mental health agency
- any phone hotline that deals with related problems (check your local yellow pages)

It is not appropriate to talk to your residents or their family members about your personal or job-related stress.

One of the best ways of managing stress in your life is to develop a plan. The plan can include nice things you will do for yourself every day and things to do in stressful situations. When you think about a plan, you first need to answer these questions:

- What are the sources of stress in my life?
- When do I most often feel stress?
- What effects of stress do I see in my life?
- What can I change to decrease the stress I feel?
- What things do I have to learn to cope with because I cannot change them?

When you have answered these questions, you will have a clearer picture of the challenges you face. Then you can come up with strategies for managing stress.

Sometimes a relaxation exercise can help you feel refreshed and relaxed in a short time. Below is a simple relaxation exercise. Try it out. See if it helps you feel more relaxed.

The Body Scan

1. Close your eyes.
2. Pay attention to your breathing and posture.
3. Be sure you are comfortable.
4. Starting at the balls of your feet, concentrate on your feet.
5. Find any tension hidden in the feet. Try to relax and release the tension.
6. Continue very slowly.
7. Take a breath between each body part.
8. Move up from the feet. Focus on and relax the legs, knees, thighs, hips, stomach, back, shoulders, neck, jaw, eyes, forehead, and scalp.
9. Take a few very deep breaths. Open your eyes.

Look back over all you have learned in this program. Your work as a nursing assistant is very important. Every day may be different and challenging. In a hundred ways every week you will offer help that only a caring person like you can give.

Value the work you have chosen to do. It is important. Your work can mean the difference between living with independence and dignity and living without. The difference you make is sometimes life versus death. Look in the face of each of your residents. Know that you are doing important work. Look in a mirror when you get home. Be proud of how you make your living.

common abbreviations

a	before	h, hr	hour	peri care	perineal care
ADL	activities of daily living	H2O	water	PPE	personal protective equipment
am, AM	morning, before noon	HBV	hepatitis B virus	p.r.n., prn	when necessary
amb	ambulatory	ht	height	q2h, q3h, etc.	every 2 hours, every 3 hours, and so on
amt	amount	hyper	above normal, too fast, rapid	q.h., qh	every hour
ap	apical	hypo	low, less than normal	q.i.d., qid	four times a day
approx.	approximately	I&O	intake and output	R	respirations, right
ax.	axillary (armpit)	inc	incontinent	reg.	regular
b.i.d.	two times a day	isol	isolation	rehab	rehabilitation
BM	bowel movement	IV	intravenous (within vein)	RN	Registered Nurse
BP, B/P	blood pressure	lab	laboratory	ROM	range of motion
BRP	bathroom privileges	lb.	pound	rt., R	right
c̄	with	LPN	Licensed Practical Nurse	s̄	without
C	Celsius	LTC	long-term care	SOB	shortness of breath
cath	catheter	LVN	Licensed Vocational Nurse	spec.	specimen
CHF	congestive heart failure	meds	medications	stat	immediately
CNA	certified nursing assistant	min	minute	STD	sexually transmitted disease
c/o	complains of	ml	milliliter	std. prec.	standard precautions
COPD	chronic obstructive pulmonary disorder	mmHg	millimeters of mercury	T, temp	temperature
CPR	cardiopulmonary resuscitation	MRSA	methicillin resistant staph aureus	TB	tuberculosis
CVA	cerebrovascular accident, stroke	N/A	not applicable	t.i.d., tid	three times a day
DNR	do not resuscitate	N.A., NA	nursing assistant	TPR	temperature, pulse, and respiration
DON	director of nursing	NKA	no known allergies	U/A, u/a	urinalysis
Dx, dx	diagnosis	PO	nothing by mouth	URI	upper respiratory infection
ER	emergency room	O2	oxygen	UTI	urinary tract infection
exam	examination	OBRA	Omnibus Budget Reconciliation Act	v.s., VS	vital signs
F	Fahrenheit or female	OOB	out of bed	w/c, W/C	wheelchair
FF	force fluids	oz.	ounce	wt.	weight
fl, fld	fluid	p̄	after		
ft	foot				

glossary

Abduction: moving a body part away from the body.

Abuse: purposely causing physical, mental, or emotional pain or injury to someone.

Activities of Daily Living (ADLs): personal care tasks a person does every day to care for him- or herself; include bathing, dressing, caring for teeth and hair, toileting, eating and drinking, and moving around.

Activity Therapy: therapy for people with Alzheimer's disease that uses activities to prevent boredom and frustration.

Acute: an illness that has severe symptoms.

Acute care: care performed in hospitals and ambulatory surgical centers.

Adaptive devices: special equipment that helps a person who is ill or disabled to perform ADLs; also called assistive devices.

Adduction: moving a body part toward the body.

Adult daycare: care given at a facility during daytime hours; generally for people who need some help but are not seriously ill or disabled.

Advance directives: documents that allow people to choose what kind of medical care they wish to have if they are unable to make those decisions themselves.

Affected side: a weakened side from a stroke or injury; also called the "weaker" or "involved" side.

Ageism: prejudice toward, stereotyping of, and/or discrimination against older persons or the elderly.

Airborne Precautions: used for diseases that can be transmitted through the air after being expelled.

Ambulation: walking.

Amputation: removal of some or all of a body part.

Angina pectoris: chest pain.

Anxiety: uneasiness or fear, often about a situation or condition.

Apathy: a lack of interest.

Aphasia: the inability to speak or to speak clearly.

Asepsis: term meaning that no infection is present.

Aspiration: the inhalation of food or drink into the lungs; can cause pneumonia or death.

Assault: when a person feels fearful that he will be touched without his permission.

Assisted living: facilities where residents live who need some assistance; they do not usually require skilled care.

Assistive devices: special equipment that helps a person who is ill or disabled to perform ADLs; also called adaptive devices.

Atrophy: the wasting away, decreasing in size, and weakening of muscles.

Autoimmune illness: condition in which the body's immune system attacks normal tissue in the body.

Battery: when a person is touched without his or her permission.

Bloodborne pathogens: microorganisms found in human blood; can cause infection and disease in humans.

Body mechanics: the way the parts of the body work together whenever a person moves.

Bony prominences: areas of the body where the bone lies close to the skin.

Cardiopulmonary resuscitation (CPR): medical procedures used when a person's heart or lungs have stopped working.

Care plan: a plan developed for each resident to achieve certain goals.

Care team: people with different education and experience who help care for residents.

Catastrophic reaction: overreacting to something in an unreasonable way.

Catheter: a tube used to drain urine from the bladder.

C. difficile (C. diff, clostridium difficile): a bacterial illness that can cause diarrhea and colitis; spread by spores in feces that are difficult to kill.

Centers for Disease Control and Prevention (CDC): a federal government agency that issues guidelines to protect and improve health.

Chain of command: the order of authority within a facility.

Chain of infection: a way to describe how disease is transmitted from one living being to another.

Charting: writing down information.

Chronic: refers to the fact that a disease or condition is long-term or long-lasting.

Clichés: phrases that are used over and over again and do not really mean anything.

Closed bed: a bed completely made with the bedspread and blankets in place.

Cognition: the ability to think logically and quickly.

Combative: violent or hostile behavior.

Combustion: the process of burning.

Communication: the process of exchanging information with others.

Compassionate: caring, concerned, empathetic, and understanding.

Condom catheter: an external catheter that has an attachment on the end that fits onto the penis; also called a Texas catheter.

Confidentiality: keeping private things private.

Confusion: the inability to think clearly.

Conscientious: always trying to do one's best.

Considerate: being understanding of residents' feelings and privacy.

Constipation: the difficult and often painful elimination of a hard, dry stool.

Constrict: to close.

Contact Precautions: used when a resident is at risk of transmitting or contracting a microorganism from touching an infected object or person.

Contractures: the permanent and often painful stiffening of a joint and muscle.

Cultural diversity: the variety of people living and working together in the world.

Culture: a system of behaviors people learn from the people they grow up and live with.

Dangle: to sit up with the feet over the side of the bed to regain balance.

Defense mechanisms: unconscious behaviors used to release tension or cope with stress.

Dehydration: a serious condition in which there is not enough fluid in the body.

Delusions: believing things that are not true.

Dementia: a serious loss of mental abilities such as thinking, remembering, reasoning, and communicating.

Dentures: artificial teeth.

Dependable: being on time and helping others when they need it.

Diabetes: a condition in which the pancreas does not produce enough insulin; causes problems with circulation and can damage vital organs.

Diagnosis: a medical condition.

Diastolic: phase when the heart relaxes.

Diet cards: cards that list the resident's name and information about special diets, allergies, likes and dislikes, and other instructions.

Digestion: the process of breaking down food so that it can be absorbed into the cells.

Dilate: to widen.

Disinfection: measure used to decrease the spread of pathogens and disease by destroying pathogens.

Disorientation: confusion about time or place.

Diuretics: drugs that reduce fluid in the body.

Domestic violence: abuse by spouses or intimate partners.

Dorsiflexion: bending backward.

Double-bagging: putting waste in a trash bag, closing it, and putting the first bag in a second, clean trash bag and closing it.

Draw sheets: turning sheets that are placed under residents who are unable to assist with turning, lifting, or moving up in bed.

Droplet Precautions: used when the disease-causing microorganism does not stay suspended in the air and travels only short distances after being expelled.

Dysphagia: difficulty swallowing.

Edema: swelling caused by excess fluid in body tissues.

Elimination: the process of expelling solid wastes that are not absorbed into the cells.

Emotional lability: laughing or crying without any reason, or when it is inappropriate.

Empathy: being able to enter into the feelings of others.

Enema: a specific amount of water flowed into the colon to eliminate stool.

Ergonomics: the practice of designing equipment and work tasks to suit the worker's abilities.

Ethics: the knowledge of right and wrong.

Expiration: exhaling air out of the lungs.

Extension: straightening a body part.

False imprisonment: the unlawful restraint of someone which affects the person's freedom of movement; includes both the threat of being physically restrained and actually being physically restrained.

Fecal impaction: a hard stool stuck in the rectum that cannot be expelled.

Financial abuse: stealing, taking advantage of, or improperly using the money, property, or other assets of another.

First aid: care given in an emergency before trained medical professionals can take over.

Flammable: easily ignited and capable of burning quickly.

Flexion: bending a body part.

Fluid balance: maintaining equal input and output, or taking in and eliminating equal amounts of fluid.

Fluid overload: a condition in which the body is unable to handle the amount of fluid consumed.

Force fluids: a medical order for a person to drink more fluids.

Fowler's: position with the person partially reclined.

Fracture: a broken bone.

Fracture pan: a bedpan used for residents who cannot assist with raising their hips onto a regular bedpan.

Gait: manner of walking.

Gastrostomy: an opening in the stomach and the abdomen.

Gestational diabetes: a condition in which pregnant women who have never had diabetes before have high blood sugar levels during pregnancy.

Glands: structures that secrete fluids.

Hallucinations: seeing or hearing things that are not there.

Hand hygiene: handwashing with soap and water and using alcohol-based hand rubs.

Health Insurance Portability and Accountability Act (HIPAA): a law that requires health information be kept private and secure; organizations must take special steps to protect health information.

Hemiparesis: weakness on one side of the body.

Hemiplegia: paralysis on one side of the body, weakness, or loss of movement.

Hepatitis: the inflammation of the liver caused by different viruses.

Hoarding: collecting and putting things away in a guarded way.

Home care: care provided in a person's home.

Homeostasis: the name for the condition in which all of the body's systems are working their best.

Hormones: chemicals that control numerous body functions.

Hospice: care for individuals who have six months or less to live; provides physical and emotional care and comfort.

Hypertension: high blood pressure.

Incident: an accident or an unexpected event during the course of care.

Incontinence: the inability to control the bladder or bowels.

Indwelling catheter: a catheter that stays in the bladder for a period of time.

Infection control: set of methods used to control and prevent the spread of disease.

Inflammation: swelling.

Informed consent: the process in which a person, with the help of his doctor, makes informed decisions about his health care.

Inspiration: breathing air into the lungs.

Insulin: a hormone that converts glucose, or natural sugar, into energy for the body.

Intake: the fluid a person consumes.

Intravenous (IV): into a vein.

Involuntary seclusion: confinement or separation from others in a certain area; done without consent or against one's will.

Lateral: position with person on his or her side.

Laws: rules set by the government to protect the people and to help them live peacefully together.

Liability: a legal term that means someone can be held responsible for harming someone else.

Localized infection: an infection limited to a specific part of the body; the infection has local symptoms.

Logrolling: moving a person as a unit, without disturbing the alignment of the body.

Long-term care (LTC): care for persons who require 24-hour care and assistance.

Masturbation: to touch or rub sexual organs in order to give oneself or another person sexual pleasure.

Menopause: the stopping of menstrual periods.

Metabolism: the body's physical and chemical processes.

Methicillin-Resistant Staphylococcus Aureus (MRSA): an infectious disease caused by bacteria that are resistant to many antibiotics.

Microorganism: a tiny living thing always present in the environment; not visible to the eye without a microscope.

Modified diet: a special diet for people who have certain illnesses; also called special or therapeutic diet.

Nasogastric tube: a special feeding tube that is inserted into the nose going to the stomach.

Neglect: failing to provide needed care.

Negligence: the failure to provide the proper care for a resident, resulting in unintended injury.

Nonverbal communication: communication without using words.

Non-weight bearing (NWB): the inability to support any weight on one or both legs.

Nosocomial infection: an infection acquired in a hospital or other healthcare facility; also known as hospital-acquired infection (HAI).

Nutrition: how the body uses food to maintain health.

Objective information: information based on what is seen, heard, touched, or smelled.

OBRA (Omnibus Budget Reconciliation Act): law passed by the federal government that established minimum standards for nursing assistant training.

Obsessive compulsive disorder: disorder in which a person uses obsessive behavior to cope with anxiety.

Obstructed airway: a condition in which a person has something blocking the tube through which air enters the lungs.

Occupied bed: a bed made while a person is in the bed.

Ombudsman: a legal advocate for residents who visits the facility, listens to residents, and decides what course of action to take if there is a problem.

Open bed: folding the linen down to the foot of the bed.

Oral care: care of the mouth, teeth, and gums.

OSHA (The Occupational Safety and Health Administration): a federal government agency that makes rules to protect workers from hazards on the job.

Osteoarthritis: a type of arthritis that usually affects hips and knees and joints of the fingers, thumbs, and spine.

Osteoporosis: a condition in which the bones become brittle and weak; may be due to age, lack of hormones, not enough calcium in bones, alcohol, or lack of exercise.

Ostomy: the surgical removal of a portion of the intestines.

Outpatient care: care usually provided for less than 24 hours for persons who have had treatments or surgery requiring short-term skilled care.

Output: eliminated fluid in urine, feces, and vomitus; it also includes perspiration and moisture in the air that is exhaled.

Pacing: walking back and forth in the same area.

Palliative: care that focuses on the comfort and dignity of the person, rather than on curing him or her.

Panic disorder: a disorder in which a person is terrified for no known reason.

Paraplegia: loss of function of lower body and legs.

Partial weight bearing (PWB): the ability to support some weight on one or both legs.

Pathogens: harmful microorganisms.

Pediculosis: an infestation of lice.

PEG tube: a feeding tube placed through the skin directly into the stomach.

Perineum: the area between the genitals and anus.

Perseverating: the repetition of a word, phrase, question, or activity over and over.

Personal: refers to life outside one's job, such as family, friends, and home life.

Personal protective equipment (PPE): a barrier between a person and disease.

Phantom sensation: pain or feeling from a body part that has been amputated.

Phobia: intense form of anxiety.

Physical abuse: any treatment, intentional or not, that causes harm to a person's body; includes slapping, bruising, cutting, burning, physically restraining, pushing, shoving, or rough handling.

Pillaging: taking things that belong to someone else.

Policy: a course of action that should be taken every time a certain situation occurs.

Portable commode: a chair with a toilet seat and a removable container underneath.

Positioning: helping people into positions that will be comfortable and healthy.

Postmortem care: care of the body after death.

Post-traumatic stress disorder: anxiety-related disorder caused by a traumatic experience.

Pre-diabetes: a condition in which a person's blood glucose levels are above normal but not high enough for a diagnosis of Type 2 diabetes.

Pressure points: areas of the body that bear much of its weight.

Pressure sore: a serious wound resulting from skin breakdown; also known as a bed sore or decubitus ulcer.

Procedure: a particular method, or way, of doing something.

Professional: having to do with work or a job.

Professionalism: how a person behaves when he or she is on the job.

Pronation: turning downward.

Prone: position with person lying on his or her stomach.

Prosthesis: an artificial body part.

Psychological abuse: emotionally harming a person by threatening, scaring, humiliating, intimidating, isolating, insulting, or treating him or her as a child; also includes verbal abuse.

Psychosocial needs: needs which involve social interaction, emotions, intellect, and spirituality.

Puree: to chop, blend, or grind food into a thick paste of baby food consistency.

Quadriplegia: loss of function of legs, trunk, and arms.

Radial pulse: the pulse site found on the inside of the wrist.

Range of motion (ROM) exercises: exercises that put a particular joint through its full arc of motion.

Reality Orientation: uses calendars, clocks, signs, and lists to help people with Alzheimer's disease remember who and where they are.

Rehabilitation: managed by professionals to restore a person to the highest possible level of functioning after an illness or injury.

Reminiscence Therapy: therapy for people with Alzheimer's disease that encourages talking about the past.

Reproduce: to create new human life.

Residents: the people who live in nursing homes.

Residents' Rights: numerous rights identified by the OBRA law for residents in long-term care facilities or nursing homes; purpose is to inform residents and others of their rights within these facilities and to provide an ethical code of conduct for healthcare workers.

Respiration: the process of breathing air into the lungs and exhaling air out of the lungs.

Restorative services: care used to keep a person at the level achieved by the rehabilitation team.

Restraint: a physical or chemical way to restrict voluntary movement or behavior.

Restraint alternatives: any intervention used in place of a restraint or that reduces the need for a restraint.

Restraint-free: an environment in which restraints are not used for any reason.

Restrict fluids: a medical order for a person to limit fluids.

Rheumatoid arthritis: a type of arthritis in which joints become red, swollen, and very painful, and movement is restricted.

Rotation: turning a joint.

Scalds: burns caused by hot liquids.

Scope of practice: defines the things a nursing assistant is allowed to do and how to do them correctly.

Sexual abuse: forcing a person to perform or participate in sexual acts.

Sexual harassment: any unwelcome sexual advance or behavior that creates an intimidating, hostile or offensive work environment.

Glossary

Shock: a condition in which the organs and tissues in the body do not receive adequate blood supply.

Skilled care: medically necessary care given by a skilled nurse or therapist.

Sims': position with person lying on his or her left side with one leg drawn up.

Special diet: a diet for people who have certain illnesses; also called therapeutic or modified diet.

Specimen: a sample.

Sputum: mucus coughed up from the lungs.

Sterilization: measure used to decrease the spread of pathogens and disease by destroying all microorganisms, not just pathogens.

Stoma: an artificial opening in body.

Straight catheter: a catheter that does not stay in the body and is removed immediately after urine is drained.

Stress: the state of being frightened, excited, confused, in danger, or irritated.

Stressor: something that causes stress.

Subacute care: care performed in either a hospital or a traditional nursing home.

Subjective information: information that cannot be or was not observed; based on what a person thinks or something that was reported by another that may or may not be true.

Substance abuse: the use of legal or illegal drugs, cigarettes, or alcohol in a way that harms oneself or others.

Supination: turning upward.

Supine: position with person lying flat on his or her back.

Suppository: a medication given rectally to cause a bowel movement.

Sympathy: sharing in the feelings and difficulties of others.

Systemic infection: an infection that occurs when pathogens enter the bloodstream and move throughout the body; causes general symptoms.

Systolic: phase where the heart is at work, contracting and pushing blood out of the left ventricle.

Tact: the ability to understand what is proper and appropriate when dealing with others.

Terminal illness: a disease or condition that will eventually cause death.

Therapeutic diet: a special diet for people who have certain illnesses; also called special or modified diet.

Total parenteral nutrition (TPN): a special type of feeding in which a person receives nutrients directly into the bloodstream.

Transfer belt: a belt made of canvas or other heavy material used to assist residents who are weak, unsteady, or uncoordinated; also called a gait belt.

Tuberculosis (TB): a bacterial infection that affects the lungs; causes coughing, difficulty breathing, fever, and fatigue.

Tumor: a group of abnormally growing cells.

Unoccupied bed: a bed made while no person is in the bed.

Validating: giving value to or approving.

Validation Therapy: therapy for people with Alzheimer's disease that lets them believe they live in the past or in imaginary circumstances.

Vancomycin-Resistant Enterococcus (VRE): a resistance caused by a person not taking all of a powerful antibiotic called Vancomycin.

Verbal abuse: oral or written words, pictures, or gestures that threaten, embarrass, or insult a person.

Verbal communication: written or spoken messages.

Wandering: walking aimlessly around the facility.

Workplace violence: abuse of staff by residents or other staff members; can be verbal, physical, or sexual.

index